ONCE-A-DAY

 Lēvaquin® Tablets / Injection
(levofloxacin tablets/injection)

Overpowers

Streptococcus pneumoniae *and other key pathogens*

Convenient Once-a-Day Dosing for All Mild-to-Severe Respiratory Indications

Infection	Due to	Dose	Duration
Community-acquired pneumonia	S pneumoniae, S aureus, H influenzae, H parainfluenzae, K pneumoniae, M catarrhalis, M pneumoniae, C pneumoniae, or L pneumophila	500 mg/q24h	7-14 days
Acute maxillary sinusitis	S pneumoniae, H influenzae, or M catarrhalis	500 mg/q24h	10-14 days
Acute bacterial exacerbation of chronic bronchitis	S pneumoniae, S aureus, H influenzae, H parainfluenzae, or M catarrhalis	500 mg/q24h	7 days

NOTE: Dosage adjustments are required in renally impaired patients.

◆ A low incidence of drug-related adverse events occurred in clinical trials: nausea (1.3%), diarrhea (1.1%), dizziness (0.4%), and insomnia (0.3%)

◆ In clinical trials, the overall patient drop-out rate due to adverse events was (3.4%)

The safety and efficacy of levofloxacin in pediatric patients, adolescents (under 18), pregnant women, and nursing mothers have not been established. Levofloxacin is contraindicated in persons with a history of hypersensitivity to levofloxacin, quinolone antimicrobial agents, or any other components of this product. Serious and occasionally fatal hypersensitivity and/or anaphylactic reactions have been reported in patients receiving therapy with quinolones, including levofloxacin. These reactions often occur following the first dose. The drug should be discontinued at the first appearance of a skin rash or any other sign of hypersensitivity.

Antacids containing magnesium or aluminum, as well as sucralfate, metal cations such as iron, and multivitamin preparations with zinc, or Videx®*(didanosine) chewable/buffered tablets or the pediatric powder for oral solution, should be taken at least 2 hours before or 2 hours after levofloxacin administration.

For information on Warnings, Precautions, and additional Adverse Reactions that may occur, regardless of drug relationship, please see full Prescribing Information.

*Videx is a registered trademark of Bristol-Myers Squibb Company.

Please see brief summary of Prescribing Information on adjacent page of this advertisement.

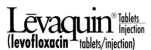

Lēvaquin® Tablets Injection
(levofloxacin tablets/injection)

Brief Summary

The following is a brief summary only. Before prescribing, see complete Prescribing Information in LEVAQUIN Injection and LEVAQUIN Tablets labeling.

CONTRAINDICATIONS

Levofloxacin is contraindicated in persons with a history of hypersensitivity to levofloxacin, quinolone antimicrobial agents, or any other components of this product.

WARNINGS

THE SAFETY AND EFFICACY OF LEVOFLOXACIN IN PEDIATRIC PATIENTS, ADOLESCENTS (UNDER THE AGE OF 18 YEARS), PREGNANT WOMEN, AND NURSING WOMEN HAVE NOT BEEN ESTABLISHED. (See **PRECAUTIONS: Pediatric Use, Pregnancy,** and **Nursing Mothers** subsections.)

In immature rats and dogs, the oral and intravenous administration of levofloxacin increased the incidence and severity of osteochondrosis. Other fluoroquinolones also produce similar erosions in the weight bearing joints and other signs of arthropathy in immature animals of various species. (See **ANIMAL PHARMACOLOGY** in full Prescribing Information.)

Convulsions and toxic psychoses have been reported in patients receiving quinolones, including levofloxacin. Quinolones may also cause increased intracranial pressure and central nervous system stimulation which may lead to tremors, restlessness, anxiety, lightheadedness, confusion, hallucinations, paranoia, depression, nightmares, insomnia, and, rarely, suicidal thoughts or acts. These reactions may occur following the first dose. If these reactions occur in patients receiving levofloxacin, the drug should be discontinued and appropriate measures instituted. As with other quinolones, levofloxacin should be used with caution in patients with a known or suspected CNS disorder that may predispose to seizures or lower the seizure threshold (e.g., severe cerebral arteriosclerosis, epilepsy) or in the presence of other risk factors that may predispose to seizures or lower the seizure threshold (e.g., certain drug therapy, renal dysfunction.) (See **PRECAUTIONS: General, Information for Patients, Drug Interactions** and **ADVERSE REACTIONS.**)

Serious and occasionally fatal hypersensitivity and/or anaphylactic reactions have been reported in patients receiving therapy with quinolones, including levofloxacin. These reactions often occur following the first dose. Some reactions have been accompanied by cardiovascular collapse, hypotension/shock, seizure, loss of consciousness, tingling, angioedema (including tongue, laryngeal, throat, or facial edema/swelling), airway obstruction (including bronchospasm, shortness of breath, and acute respiratory distress), dyspnea, urticaria, itching, and other serious skin reactions. Levofloxacin should be discontinued immediately at the first appearance of a skin rash or any other sign of hypersensitivity. Serious acute hypersensitivity reactions may require treatment with epinephrine and other resuscitative measures, including oxygen, intravenous fluids, antihistamines, corticosteroids, pressor amines, and airway management, as clinically indicated. (See **PRECAUTIONS** and **ADVERSE REACTIONS.**)

Serious and sometimes fatal events, some due to hypersensitivity, and some due to uncertain etiology, have been reported rarely in patients receiving therapy with quinolones, including levofloxacin. These events may be severe and generally occur following the administration of multiple doses. Clinical manifestations may include one or more of the following: fever, rash or severe dermatologic reactions (e.g., toxic epidermal necrolysis, Stevens-Johnson Syndrome); vasculitis; arthralgia; myalgia; serum sickness; allergic pneumonitis; interstitial nephritis; acute renal insufficiency or failure; hepatitis; jaundice; acute hepatic necrosis or failure; anemia, including hemolytic and aplastic; thrombocytopenia, including thrombotic thrombocytopenic purpura; leukopenia; agranulocytosis; pancytopenia; and/or other hematologic abnormalities. The drug should be discontinued immediately at the first appearance of a skin rash or any other sign of hypersensitivity and supportive measures instituted. (See **PRECAUTIONS: Information for Patients** and **ADVERSE REACTIONS.**)

Pseudomembranous colitis has been reported with nearly all antibacterial agents, including levofloxacin, and may range in severity from mild to life-threatening. Therefore, it is important to consider this diagnosis in patients who present with diarrhea subsequent to the administration of any antibacterial agent.

Treatment with antibacterial agents alters the normal flora of the colon and may permit overgrowth of clostridia. Studies indicate that a toxin produced by *Clostridium difficile* is one primary cause of "antibiotic-associated colitis".

After the diagnosis of pseudomembranous colitis has been established, therapeutic measures should be initiated. Mild cases of pseudomembranous colitis usually respond to drug discontinuation alone. In moderate to severe cases, consideration should be given to management with fluids and electrolytes, protein supplementation, and treatment with an antibacterial drug clinically effective against *C. difficile* colitis. (See **ADVERSE REACTIONS.**)

Ruptures of the shoulder, hand, or Achilles tendons that required surgical repair or resulted in prolonged disability have been reported in patients receiving quinolones, including levofloxacin. Levofloxacin should be discontinued if the patient experiences pain, inflammation, or rupture of a tendon. Patients should rest and refrain from exercise until the diagnosis of tendinitis or tendon rupture has been confidently excluded. Tendon rupture can occur during or after therapy with quinolones, including levofloxacin.

PRECAUTIONS

General:

Because a rapid or bolus intravenous injection may result in hypotension, LEVOFLOXACIN INJECTION SHOULD ONLY BE ADMINISTERED BY SLOW INTRAVENOUS INFUSION OVER A PERIOD OF 60 MINUTES. (See **DOSAGE AND ADMINISTRATION.**)

Although levofloxacin is more soluble than other quinolones, adequate hydration of patients receiving levofloxacin should be maintained to prevent the formation of a highly concentrated urine.

Administer levofloxacin with caution in the presence of renal insufficiency. Careful clinical observation and appropriate laboratory studies should be performed prior to and during therapy since elimination of levofloxacin may be reduced. In patients with impaired renal function (creatinine clearance ≤80 mL/min), adjustment of the dosage regimen is necessary to avoid the accumulation of levofloxacin due to decreased clearance. (See **CLINICAL PHARMACOLOGY** and **DOSAGE AND ADMINISTRATION.**)

Moderate to severe phototoxicity reactions have been observed in patients exposed to direct sunlight while receiving drugs in this class. Excessive exposure to sunlight should be avoided. However, in clinical trials with levofloxacin, phototoxicity has been observed in less than 0.1% of patients. Therapy should be discontinued if phototoxicity (e.g., a skin eruption) occurs.

As with other quinolones, levofloxacin should be used with caution in any patient with a known or suspected CNS disorder that may predispose to seizures or lower the seizure threshold (e.g., severe cerebral arteriosclerosis, epilepsy) or in the presence of other risk factors that may predispose to seizures or lower the seizure threshold (e.g., certain drug therapy, renal dysfunction). (See **WARNINGS** and **Drug Interactions.**)

As with other quinolones, disturbances of blood glucose, including symptomatic hyper- and hypoglycemia, have been reported, usually in diabetic patients receiving concomitant treatment with an oral hypoglycemic agent (e.g., glyburide/glibenclamide) or with insulin. In these patients, careful monitoring of blood glucose is recommended. If a hypoglycemic reaction occurs in a patient being treated with levofloxacin, levofloxacin should be discontinued immediately and appropriate therapy should be initiated immediately. (See **Drug Interactions** and **ADVERSE REACTIONS.**)

As with any potent antimicrobial drug, periodic assessment of organ system functions, including renal, hepatic, and hematopoietic, is advisable during therapy. (See **WARNINGS** and **ADVERSE REACTIONS.**)

Information for Patients:

Patients should be advised:

- to drink fluids liberally;
- that levofloxacin may cause neurologic adverse effects (e.g., dizziness, lightheadedness) and that patients should know how they react to levofloxacin before they operate an automobile or machinery or engage in other activities requiring mental alertness and coordination. (See **WARNINGS** and **ADVERSE REACTIONS**);
- to discontinue treatment and inform their physician if they experience pain, inflammation, or rupture of a tendon, and to rest and refrain from exercise until the diagnosis of tendinitis or tendon rupture has been confidently excluded;
- that levofloxacin may be associated with hypersensitivity reactions, even following the first dose, and to discontinue the drug at the first sign of a skin rash, hives or other skin reactions, a rapid heartbeat, difficulty in swallowing or breathing, any swelling suggesting angioedema (e.g., swelling of the lips, tongue, face, tightness of the throat, hoarseness), or other symptoms of an allergic reaction. (See **WARNINGS** and **ADVERSE REACTIONS**);
- to avoid excessive sunlight or artificial ultraviolet light while receiving levofloxacin and to discontinue therapy if phototoxicity (i.e., skin eruption) occurs;
- that if they are diabetic and are being treated with insulin or an oral hypoglycemic agent and a hypoglycemic reaction occurs, they should discontinue levofloxacin and consult a physician. (See **PRECAUTIONS: General** and **Drug Interactions.**)
- that convulsions have been reported in patients taking quinolones, including levofloxacin, and to notify their physician before taking this drug if there is a history of this condition.
- that if therapy with oral levofloxacin is initiated, then (1) antacids containing magnesium, or aluminum, as well as sucralfate, metal cations such as iron, and multivitamin preparations with zinc or Videx®, (Didanosine), chewable/buffered tablets or the pediatric powder for oral solution should be taken at least two hours before or two hours after levofloxacin administration. (See **Drug Interactions**); and (2) oral levofloxacin can be taken without regard to meals.

Drug Interactions:

Antacids, Sucralfate, Metal Cations, Multivitamins

LEVAQUIN Injection: There are no data concerning an interaction of **Intravenous** quinolones with **oral** antacids, sucralfate, multivitamins, Videx®, (Didanosine), or metal cations. However, no quinolone should be co-administered with any solution containing multivalent cations, e.g., magnesium, through the same intravenous line. (See **DOSAGE AND ADMINISTRATION.**)

LEVAQUIN Tablets: While the chelation by divalent cations is less marked than with other quinolones, concurrent administration of LEVAQUIN Tablets with antacids containing magnesium, or aluminum, as well as sucralfate, metal cations such as iron, and multivitamins preparations with zinc may interfere with the gastrointestinal absorption of levofloxacin, resulting in systemic levels considerably lower than desired. Tablets with antacids containing magnesium, aluminum, as well as sucralfate, metal cations such as iron, and multivitamins preparations with zinc or Videx®, (Didanosine) chewable/buffered tablets or the pediatric powder for oral solution may substantially interfere with the gastrointestinal absorption of levofloxacin, resulting in systemic levels considerably lower than desired. These agents should be taken at least two hours before or two hours after levofloxacin administration.

Theophylline: No significant effect of levofloxacin on the plasma concentrations, AUC, and other disposition parameters for theophylline was detected in a clinical study involving 14 healthy volunteers. Similarly, no apparent effect of theophylline on levofloxacin absorption and disposition was observed. However, concomitant administration of other quinolones with theophylline has resulted in prolonged elimination half-life, elevated serum theophylline levels, and a subsequent increase in the risk of theophylline-related adverse reactions in the patient population. Therefore, theophylline levels should be closely monitored and appropriate dosage adjustments made when levofloxacin is co-administered. Adverse reactions, including seizures, may occur with or without an elevation in serum theophylline levels. (See **WARNINGS** and **PRECAUTIONS: General.**)

Warfarin: No significant effect of levofloxacin on the peak plasma concentrations, AUC, and other disposition parameters for R- and S- warfarin was detected in a clinical study involving healthy volunteers. No significant change in prothrombin time was noted in the presence of levofloxacin. Similarly, no apparent effect of warfarin on levofloxacin absorption and disposition was observed. However, since some quinolones have been reported to enhance the effects of oral anticoagulant warfarin or its derivatives in the patient population, the prothrombin time or other suitable coagulation test should be closely monitored if a quinolone antimicrobial is administered concomitantly with warfarin or its derivatives.

Cyclosporine: No significant effect of levofloxacin on the peak plasma concentrations, AUC, and other disposition parameters for cyclosporine was detected in a clinical study involving healthy volunteers. However, elevated serum levels of cyclosporine have been reported in the patient population when co-administered with some other quinolones. Levofloxacin C_{max} and k_e were slightly lower while T_{max} and $t_{1/2}$ were slightly longer in the presence of cyclosporine than those observed in other studies without concomitant medication. The differences, however, are not considered to be clinically significant. Therefore, no dosage adjustment is required for levofloxacin or cyclosporine when administered concomitantly.

Digoxin: No significant effect of levofloxacin on the peak plasma concentrations, AUC, and other disposition parameters for digoxin was detected in a clinical study involving healthy volunteers. Levofloxacin absorption and disposition kinetics were similar in the presence or absence of digoxin. Therefore, no dosage adjustment for levofloxacin or digoxin is required when administered concomitantly.

Probenecid and Cimetidine: No significant effect of probenecid or cimetidine on the rate and extent of levofloxacin absorption was observed in a clinical study involving healthy volunteers. The AUC and $t_{1/2}$ of levofloxacin were 27-38% and 30% higher, respectively, while CL/F and CL_R were 21-35% lower during concomitant treatment with probenecid or cimetidine compared to levofloxacin alone. Although these differences were statistically significant, the changes were not high enough to warrant dosage adjustment for levofloxacin when probenecid or cimetidine is co-administered.

Non-steroidal anti-inflammatory drugs: The concomitant administration of a non-steroidal anti-inflammatory drug with a quinolone, including levofloxacin, may increase the risk of CNS stimulation and convulsive seizures. (See **WARNINGS** and **PRECAUTIONS: General.**)

Antidiabetic agents: Disturbances of blood glucose, including hyperglycemia and hypoglycemia, have been reported in patients treated concomitantly with quinolones and an antidiabetic agent. Therefore, careful monitoring of blood glucose is recommended when these agents are co-administered.

Carcinogenesis, Mutagenesis, Impairment of Fertility:

In a long term carcinogenicity study in rats, levofloxacin exhibited no carcinogenic or tumorigenic potential following daily dietary administration for 2 years; the highest dose was 2 or 10 times the recommended human dose based on surface area or body weight, respectively.

Levofloxacin was not mutagenic in the following assays; Ames bacterial mutation assay (*S. typhimurium* and *E. coli*), CHO/HGPRT forward mutation assay, mouse micronucleus test, mouse dominant lethal test, rat unscheduled DNA synthesis assay, and the mouse sister chromatid exchange assay. It was positive in the *in vitro* chromosomal aberration (CHL cell line) and sister chromatid exchange (CHL/IU cell line) assays.

Levofloxacin caused no impairment of fertility or reproductive performance in rats at oral doses as high as 360 mg/kg/day (2124 mg/m^2), corresponding to 3.0 or 18 times the recommended maximum human dose based on surface area or body weight, respectively, and intravenous doses as high as 100 mg/kg/day (590 mg/m^2), corresponding to 1.0 or 5 times the recommended maximum human dose based on surface area or body weight, respectively.

Pregnancy: Teratogenic Effects. Pregnancy Category C.

Levofloxacin was not teratogenic in rats at oral doses as high as 810 mg/kg/day (4779 mg/m^2), which corresponds to 14 or 82 times the recommended maximum human dose based on surface area or body weight, respectively, or at intravenous doses as high as 160 mg/kg/day (944 mg/m^2) corresponding to 2.7 or 16 times the recommended maximum human dose based on surface area or body weight, respectively. Doses equivalent to 26 or 81 times the recommended maximum human dose of levofloxacin (based on surface area or body weight, respectively) caused decreased fetal body weight and increased fetal mortality in rats when administered orally at 810 mg/kg/day (8910 mg/m^2). No teratogenicity was observed when rabbits were dosed orally as high as 50 mg/kg/day (550 mg/m^2) which corresponds to 1.6 or 5.0 times the recommended maximum human dose based on surface area or body weight, respectively, or when dosed intravenously as high as 25 mg/kg/day (275 mg/m^2), corresponding to 0.8 or 2.5 times the maximum recommended human dose based on surface area or body weight, respectively.

There are, however, no adequate and well-controlled studies in pregnant women. Levofloxacin should be used during pregnancy only if the potential benefit justifies the potential risk to the fetus. (See **WARNINGS.**)

Nursing Mothers:

Levofloxacin has not been measured in human milk. Based upon data from ofloxacin, it can be presumed that levofloxacin will be excreted in human milk. Because of the potential for serious adverse reactions from levofloxacin in nursing infants, a decision should be made whether to discontinue nursing or to discontinue the drug, taking into account the importance of the drug to the mother.

Pediatric Use:

Safety and effectiveness in pediatric patients and adolescents below the age of 18 years have not been established. Quinolones, including levofloxacin, cause arthropathy and osteochondrosis in juvenile animals of several species. (See **WARNINGS.**)

ADVERSE REACTIONS

The incidence of drug-related adverse reactions in patients during Phase 3 clinical trials conducted in North America was 6.2%. Among patients receiving levofloxacin therapy, 3.4% discontinued levofloxacin therapy due to adverse experiences.

In clinical trials, the following events were considered likely to be drug-related in patients receiving levofloxacin:
nausea 1.3%, diarrhea 1.1%, vaginitis 0.7%, pruritus 0.5%, abdominal pain 0.4%, dizziness 0.4%, flatulence 0.4%, rash 0.4%, dyspepsia 0.3%, genital moniliasis 0.3%, insomnia 0.3%, taste perversion 0.2%, vomiting 0.2%, anorexia 0.1%, anxiety 0.1%, constipation 0.1%, edema 0.1%, fatigue 0.1%, fungal infection 0.1%, headache 0.1%, increased sweating 0.1%, leukorrhea 0.1%, malaise 0.1%, nervousness 0.1%, sleep disorders 0.1%, tremor 0.1%, urticaria 0.1%.

In clinical trials, the following events occurred in >3% of patients regardless of drug relationship:
nausea 7.1%, headache 6.4%, diarrhea 5.6%, injection site reaction 5.6%, insomnia 4.0%.

In clinical trials, the following events occurred in 1 to 3% of patients, regardless of drug relationship:
constipation 2.9%, dizziness 2.9%, injection site pain 2.7%, abdominal pain 2.6%, dyspepsia 2.5%, vomiting 2.2%, rash 1.7%, flatulence 1.6%, vaginitis 1.6%, pruritus 1.5%, fatigue 1.3%, injection site inflammation 1.5%, back pain 1.2%, pain 1.2%, chest pain 1.1%, pharyngitis 1.1%, rhinitis 1.1%, taste perversion 1.0%.

In clinical trials, the following events occurred in 0.5 to less than 1% of patients, regardless of drug relationship:
anorexia, anxiety, arthralgia, coughing, dry mouth, dyspnea, ear disorder (not otherwise specified), edema, fever, fungal infection, genital pruritus, increased sweating, skin disorder, somnolence.

In clinical trials, the following events, of potential medical importance, occurred at a rate of less than 0.5% regardless of drug relationship:
abnormal coordination, abnormal dreaming, abnormal hepatic function, abnormal platelets, abnormal renal function, abnormal vision, acute renal failure, aggravated diabetes mellitus, aggressive reaction, agitation, anemia, angina pectoris, ARDS, arrhythmia, arthritis, arthrosis, asthenia, asthma, atrial fibrillation, bradycardia, cardiac arrest, cardiac failure, carcinoma, cerebrovascular disorder, cholelithiasis, circulatory failure, coma, confusion, conjunctivitis, convulsions (seizures), coronary thrombosis, dehydration, delirium, depression, diplopia, dysphagia, ejaculation failure, embolism (blood clot), emotional lability, epistaxis, erythema nodosum, face edema, gastroenteritis, genital moniliasis, G.I. hemorrhage, granulocytopenia, haematuria, haemoptysis, hallucination, heart block, hepatic coma, hyperglycemia, hyperkalemia, hyperkinesia, hypertension, hypertonia, hypoaesthesia, hypoglycemia, hypokalemia, hypotension, hypoxia, impaired concentration, impotence, increased LDH, involuntary muscle contractions, jaundice, leukocytosis, leukopenia, lymphadenopathy, malaise, manic reaction, mental deficiency, muscle weakness, myalgia, myocardial infarction, nervousness, palpitation, pancreatitis, paraesthesia, paralysis, paranoia, parosmia, phlebitis, pleural effusion, postural hypotension, pseudomembranous colitis, purpura, respiratory insufficiency, rhabdomyolysis, rigors, skin exfoliation, skin ulceration, sleep disorders, speech disorder, stupor, substernal chest pain, supraventricular tachycardia, syncope, synovitis, tachycardia, tendinitis, thrombocytopenia, tinnitus, tongue edema, tremor, urticaria, ventricular fibrillation, vertigo, weight decrease, WBC abnormal (not otherwise specified), withdrawl syndrome.

In clinical trials using multiple-dose therapy, ophthalmologic abnormalities, including cataracts and multiple punctate lenticular opacities, have been noted in patients undergoing treatment with other quinolones. The relationship of the drugs to these events is not presently established.

Crystalluria and cylindruria have been reported with other quinolones.

The following laboratory abnormalities appeared in 2.1 to 2.3% of patients receiving levofloxacin. It is not known whether these abnormalities were caused by the drug or the underlying condition being treated.

Blood Chemistry: decreased glucose
Hematology: decreased lymphocytes

Post-Marketing Adverse Reactions:

Additional adverse events reported from worldwide post-marketing experience with levofloxacin include:
allergic pneumonitis, anaphylactic shock, anaphylactoid reaction, dysphonia, abnormal EEG, encephalopathy, eosinophilia, erythema multiforme, hemolytic anemia, multi-system organ failure, Stevens-Johnson Syndrome, tendon rupture, vasodilation.

ORTHO-McNEIL PHARMACEUTICAL, INC.
Raritan, New Jersey, USA 08869
U.S. Patent No. 4,382,892 and U.S. Patent No. 5,053,407. 633-10-811-3B

Revised August 1998 635-10-287-3B

ORTHO-McNEIL

Ortho-McNeil Pharmaceutical, Inc.
Raritan, NJ 08869-0602

DAIICHI

©OMP 1999 02R4216A 1/99

An Atlas of
LUNG INFECTIONS

THE ENCYCLOPEDIA OF VISUAL MEDICINE SERIES

An Atlas of
LUNG INFECTIONS

J. F. Costello

Department of Thoracic Medicine
King's College School of Medicine & Dentistry
London

D. E. Saunders

St. George's Hospital Medical School
London

and

J. Philpott-Howard

Dulwich Public Health Laboratory and Medical Microbiology
King's College School of Medicine & Dentistry
London

With a Foreword by
Philip C. Hopewell, MD

Chief, Division of Pulmonary & Critical Care Medicine,
San Francisco General Hospital
and
Professor of Medicine, University of California
San Francisco

The Parthenon Publishing Group
International Publishers in Medicine, Science & Technology

NEW YORK   LONDON

British Library Cataloguing-in-Publication Data
Costello, J.F.
   Atlas of Lung Infections
   I. Title
   616.24

ISBN 1-85070-456-2

Library of Congress Cataloging-in-Publication Data
Costello, J.F. (John Francis). 1944–
      An atlas of lung infections / J.F. Costello, D.E. Saunders, and
   J. Philpott-Howard.
         p.   cm.–(The encyclopedia of visual medicine series)
      Includes bibliographical references and index.
      I. Respiratory infections–Atlases.   I. Saunders, D.E.
   II. Philpott-Howard, J.   III. Title.   IV. Title: Lung infections.
   V. Series.
      [DNLM: I. Lung Diseases–diagnosis–atlases.
      WF 17 C841a 1995]
   RC740.C67   1995
   616.2'4075–dc20
   DNLM/DLC
   for Library of Congress   96-2478
                                                              CIP

Published in the UK and Europe by
The Parthenon Publishing Group Limited
Casterton Hall, Carnforth
Lancs. LA6 2LA

Published in the USA by
The Parthenon Publishing Group Inc.
One Blue Hill Plaza,
PO Box 1564, Pearl River,
New York 10965, USA

Copyright © 1996 Parthenon Publishing Group Ltd

Reprinted 1999

*No part of this book may be reproduced in any form without
permission from the publishers, except for the quotation of brief
passages for the purposes of review.*

Composition by Ryburn Publishing Services,
Keele University, Staffordshire, England
Printed and bound by TG Hostench S.A., Spain

Contents

The Encyclopedia of Visual Medicine Series

Titles currently planned in this series include:

An Atlas of Oncology

An Atlas of Hypertension

An Atlas of Common Diseases

An Atlas of Osteoporosis

An Atlas of the Menopause

An Atlas of Contraception

An Atlas of Endometriosis

An Atlas of Ultrasonography in Obstetrics and Gynecology

An Atlas of Practical Radiology

An Atlas of Psoriasis

An Atlas of Trauma Management

An Atlas of Lung Infections

An Atlas of Transvaginal Color Doppler

An Atlas of Infective Endocarditis

An Atlas of Rheumatology

An Atlas of Epilepsy

An Atlas of Differential Diagnosis in HIV Disease

An Atlas of Practical Dermatology

An Atlas of Laser Operative Laparoscopy and Hysteroscopy

An Atlas of Atherosclerosis

An Atlas of Eye Diseases

An Atlas of Cutaneous Growths

An Atlas of Myocardial Infarction

An Atlas of Diabetes Mellitus

Foreword

Much of the information upon which diagnoses and approaches to treatment are based is derived from visual assessments – observation of patients themselves, interpretations of radiographic studies, and microscopic and bacteriological examinations of secretions and tissues, to name a few. Yet, in spite of our heavy reliance on visual data, standard textbooks rarely contain sufficient examples to be truly useful in this regard, and words cannot convey the descriptions adequately. This *Atlas of Lung Infections* is a welcome departure from traditional textbooks and will be an important resource for clinicians who are involved in the care of patients with lung diseases.

Infections of the lower respiratory tract are the cause of substantial morbidity and mortality and are included in the differential diagnosis of many respiratory disorders. Thus, these infections occupy a considerable proportion of working hours for pulmonologists, internists and specialists in infectious diseases. Each of the three major clinical categories of lower respiratory tract infections, community-acquired, and hospital-acquired pneumonias and pneumonias in immunocompromised hosts, has distinct although overlapping lists of possible etiological agents. Community-acquired pneumonias present diagnostic difficulty because of the high proportion caused by non-bacterial pathogens. Particularly problematic are hospital-acquired pneumonias. This latter category of lung infections is difficult to detect when superimposed on a background of pre-existing lung disease and difficult to treat specifically because identification of the etiological agent is not easily accomplished. Moreover, hospital-acquired infections impose a significant increase in inpatient stays and in the likelihood of death. Respiratory infection in immunocompromised hosts is an increasingly important category of illness. In such patients, the differential diagnosis is broad and includes both opportunistic and non-opportunistic pathogens.

For all three categories of infection, rapid and specific diagnoses provide the clinician with the information necessary to begin appropriate chemotherapy. In this context 'appropriate chemotherapy' infers that the agents used are not only effective but also have the narrowest possible spectrum. The pictorial information and accompanying descriptions contained in this Atlas will be highly useful in enabling clinicians to make accurate diagnoses by collecting relevant specimens and obtaining the highest yield studies. Moreover, the correlations among the clinical, radiographic and microbiological features of an infection will facilitate the interaction between clinicians and microbiology laboratories so as to make for more effective and efficient utilization of laboratory tests.

Philip C. Hopewell, MD
Chief, Division of Pulmonary & Critical Care Medicine,
San Francisco General Hospital
Professor of Medicine, University of California,
San Francisco

Introduction

The aim of this Atlas is to provide trainees in many areas of hospital and community medicine with a readily accessible guide to the presentation and diagnosis of infections of the lower respiratory tract. Each of the four main sections provides a review of the most common infections, and some rarer diseases. Radiographs are accompanied by the relevant micro-biological or histological preparation in order to give the reader a complete picture of the diagnostic approach to the infection; many examining boards in general medicine and other relevant specialties expect trainees to recognize and understand these laboratory procedures. We hope that the Atlas will also prove useful for clinicians who may only occasionally encounter some of the infections we have illustrated.

Acknowledgements

The authors wish to acknowledge the invaluable assistance of the following:

Mr Paul Bracken, Dr David Dance, Mr Ken Davies, Dr Edward Gane, Dr Philip Gishen, Dr Robert Hill, Dr Julian Hodgson, Dr David Hughes, Dr John Karani, Dr Pauline Kane, Dr Richard Kent, Dr Nigel Marchbank, Professor John Moxham, Dr Ghulam Mufti, Professor John Price, Dr John Ramage, Dr John Salisbury, Mr Ron Senkus, Dr Sheena Sutherland, Dr Alan Wilson, Professor Phillip Hopewell, and Gower Medical Publishing.

Section 1   A Review of Lung Infections

Developments in the diagnosis and management of respiratory infections

Introduction

Respiratory tract infection is a common cause of death in children world-wide and accounts for at least one-third of all adult deaths. In addition, there is an inestimable childhood and adult morbidity with a huge impact on the health, work and social economy of every nation. In developed countries, medical consultations for mild to moderate respiratory tract infection can account for 50% of the physician's workload, whilst the specific diagnosis and management of severe pneumonia continue to present considerable difficulties in the hospitalized patient.

Despite recent advances in this field, one of the most challenging aspects of respiratory tract infection is the development of methods for a rapid and specific diagnosis. For many mild to moderate community-acquired respiratory infections, particularly those due to viruses, efforts to identify the pathogen are rarely made, since laboratory techniques are often labor-intensive and expensive, and there are few effective therapies. Even in patients with lung infection, rapid diagnostic methods for specific pathogens are few and serological studies are rarely of benefit in the acute management of the infection; also, conventional microbiological techniques may yield a pathogen in only one-third to one-half of cases of pneumonia. Despite these problems, the combined efforts of the clinician and laboratory can lead to a satisfactory outcome in the great majority of pulmonary infections.

Rapid advances in the management of respiratory tract infections should be forthcoming in the next decade. Clearly, researchers must aim to provide tests which are sensitive, specific, rapid, inexpensive and readily performed by the majority of laboratories, at the bedside or in the clinic. Such diagnostic advances must, of course, be accompanied by the development of specific oral or parenteral therapies to improve morbidity and reduce patient-related costs. Antimicrobial development has lately focused on drugs of particular relevance to respiratory disease, such as macrolides, azalides, quinolones and oral broad-spectrum β-lactam antibiotics. The development of immune modifiers such as anti-tumor necrosis factor and anti-interleukins will also have a significant impact, particularly on hospital respiratory medicine.

Apart from the laboratory diagnosis of respiratory infections, the clinician is assisted by progress in other fields. Improved radiological techniques, such as computerized tomography, magnetic resonance imaging, radionucleide scanning and fluoroscopy-guided biopsy, have had a major impact on respiratory medicine. Improved flexible bronchoscopes and growing readiness to perform bronchoscopy have also increased the use of these techniques and introduced a broader base of experience amongst respiratory physicians in training. In many centers, bronchial lavage with or without transbronchial biopsy has virtually replaced the potentially hazardous methods of open lung biopsy and transtracheal aspiration. These methods are especially applicable to the ever-increasing population of patients with acquired immune deficiency syndrome (AIDS) or other immune deficiencies which place them at risk of severe and life-threatening respiratory infection.

The diagnosis of respiratory tract infection

Clinical assessment
Although time-honored methods of obtaining the patient's history and performing an examination need no description, the importance of eliciting specific information and clinical signs, when evaluating the patient with lower respiratory infection, cannot be overemphasized. In particular, the following must be noted:

(1) *History*
   (a) Pre-existing pulmonary and systemic disease;
   (b) Recent immunosuppressive and antimicrobial therapy;
   (c) Animal (particularly avian) exposure;
   (d) Sexual history, drug abuse and other risk factors for human immunodeficiency virus (HIV);
   (e) Occupational history;
   (f) Overseas travel and ethnicity;
   (g) Tuberculosis contact.

(2) *Examination*
   (a) Lymphadenopathy;
   (b) Evidence of drug self-injection;
   (c) Dentition and presence of oral *Candida*;
   (d) Skin rash;
   (e) Fundal examination;
   (f) Respiratory rate, particularly in children;
   (g) Macroscopic appearance of sputum.

Microbiological examination of sputum and other samples
Obtaining specimens Specimens for microbiology should be taken before antibiotics are started, if at all possible, and sent in a secure leakproof container, approved by the laboratory, with a minimum of delay.

Although sputum samples are frequently sent to the laboratory, they may be of little value. This is because samples are often salivary; adequate expectoration of bronchial secretions has not taken place. Immunocompromised patients may produce few respiratory secretions and chest physiotherapy may be required to obtain a specimen; in some instances the patient can be asked to inhale a saline aerosol to induce coughing and expectoration. If these methods fail, and particularly if the patient is rapidly declining or seriously ill, the clinician may choose to perform one or more of the following techniques in order to provide material for microscopy and culture:

(1) Flexible bronchoscopy with saline lavage, protected brushing and/or transbronchial biopsy;

(2) Percutaneous aspiration or biopsy of focal pulmonary lesions with or without fluoroscopy guidance;

(3) Transtracheal aspirate;

(4) Open lung biopsy;

(5) Pleural aspirate and biopsy, in the presence of a pleural effusion.

Other samples may be of value in the diagnosis of pulmonary infections, in particular: blood cultures; urine or serum for the detection of bacterial antigens by latex agglutination or countercurrent immunoelectrophoresis; nasopharyngeal washings or swabs in viral transport medium; feces (or a rectal swab in viral transport medium); feces and special blood cultures for *Mycobacterium avium* complex; and serum for a wide range of complement fixation tests, ELISAs and agglutination tests. Serum is also useful for cryptococcal antigen and *Candida* antigen testing in selected cases. Upper airway swabs may sometimes reflect lower respiratory flora, particularly in neutropenic patients when *Aspergillus* spp. or large numbers of opportunist Gram-negative aerobes may be cultured.

Microscopy   The most commonly used microscopic methods are the Gram stain, which is particularly useful for the examination of purulent sputum in acute pneumonia, or for the examination of saline lung washings and biopsies, and the Ziehl–Neelsen (or auramine) stain for acid-alcohol fast bacilli in any sample. In addition, several staining methods may be of value in selected patients, and routinely for biopsy or lavage samples:

(1) Wet preparation with lactophenol cotton blue for fungal hyphae;

(2) Modified Giemsa or Grocott silver stain for *Pneumocystis carinii*;

(3) A modified Ziehl–Neelsen stain for *Nocardia* spp. and *Actinomyces*;

(4) Histological stains for specific pathology including intranuclear inclusion bodies (e.g. cytomegalovirus), periodic acid-Schiff for fungal elements, and miscellaneous stains for neoplastic cells and other histological features;

(5) Examination for parasites, e.g. *Paragonimus*; and larvae of *Strongyloides stercoralis* or *Ascaris lumbricoides*.

The interpretation of wet-mounted or stained preparations requires caution. Direct microscopy is insensitive – bacteria are unlikely to be seen, even with careful examination of the film, unless about 10^5 organisms per ml of fluid are present. Also, contaminating flora, such as pharyngeal streptococci, may be visible in sputum and occasionally in bronchial washings. In contrast, large numbers of capsulate diplococci, clustering Gram-positive cocci or numerous Gram-negative rods seen in such specimens, in the appropriate clinical setting, can be useful indicators of infection with pneumococci, staphylococci or aerobic Gram-negative rods, respectively.

Because of the limitations of some types of direct microscopy, other methods have been applied using monoclonal antibodies for viruses and bacteria; the most frequently used technique is direct immunofluorescent staining for viruses such as respiratory syncytial virus, influenza virus, and herpesviruses. *Chlamydia trachomatis*, *Legionella pneumophila* and *Pneumocystis carinii* can also be detected in this way. Other methods such as immunoperoxidase staining have been developed for *Pneumocystis carinii* and *Haemophilus influenzae*.

Some workers have examined bronchoalveolar lavage cell populations in an attempt to evaluate the outcome of severity of respiratory illness in HIV patients. Patients with a higher neutrophil/lymphocyte ratio tend to have more severe disease. Although such methods are in their infancy, the rapid development and increasing sophistication of molecular, immunological and cell techniques mean that direct analysis of patient samples will provide significantly more information than is available at present to guide the clinician in patient management.

Culture   Culture of significant pathogenic microorganisms in respiratory disease provides the gold standard with which all other methods are compared, particularly rapid direct examination of samples, as outlined above, and serological tests. Because of the wide range of potential pathogens, and the significance of underlying immunosuppression in relation to lower respiratory infection, the laboratory must be provided with adequate clinical and demographic information in order to process the samples in the most appropriate manner.

There are several laboratory methods which can improve the value of specimen culture. Organisms are often unevenly distributed in viscous samples; *sputolysin* is an enzyme which breaks down mucus and permits homogenization of sputum or other viscous material, and pretreatment of sputum is now practised in many laboratories prior to inoculation of culture plates.

Quantitative culture by dilution of bronchoalveolar lavage samples can help to distinguish between contaminating pharyngeal flora or reveal small numbers of pathogens obscured by other organisms. *Culture of anaerobes* when indicated is more likely to yield delicate anaerobic organisms if pre-reduced culture plates (i.e. those held in an anaerobic atmosphere prior to inoculation) are used.

Special culture media may be inoculated, according to the clinical information available, for example:

(1) *Legionella* spp. (from bronchial washings);

(2) *Mycobacterium* spp.;

(3) Fungi;

(4) *Mycoplasma pneumoniae* (rarely undertaken); genital mycoplasmas (neonates);

(5) Anaerobes, if necrotizing pneumonia or a lung abscess is present;

(6) Herpesviruses.

Unusual pathogens encountered in diseases such as AIDS may require extended culture or specific media and incubation temperatures, particularly to facilitate growth of environmental mycobacteria and fungi. Although some laboratories culture all sputa for *Mycobacterium tuberculosis*, this practice is uncommon and a specific request must be made.

Interpretation of culture results is not always easy, particularly when the isolate is known to be part of the normal microbial flora of the upper respiratory tract. For example, in patients with chronic bronchitis, large numbers of colonizing haemophili and pneumococci are frequently cultured, even in the absence of infection, and the value of routine sputum culture in such cases is doubtful. The role of *Moraxella catarrhalis*, widely recognized as a potential pathogen, remains unclear in some patients; premature neonates may have tracheal colonization with coagulase-negative staphylococci, but in some circumstances this may represent true pulmonary infection.

Serology and other tests An increasing range of serological tests is available, and, to avoid unnecessary costs, clinicians should identify and agree upon a range of tests, in some order of priority, that are most appropriate for their patient group. Clearly, this will depend primarily on the severity of the illness, radiological appearances, and the underlying clinical disorder. For example, serological tests associated with specific organisms can be summarized as follows:

(1) *Acute community-acquired pneumonia*

  (a) *Mycoplasma pneumoniae*: complement fixation test (CFT), cold agglutinins;
  (b) *Chlamydia* spp.: CFT, microimmunofluorescence;
  (c) *Legionella* spp.: rapid micro-agglutination and immunofluorescent antibody test;
  (d) *Coxiella burnetii*: CFT;
  (e) Respiratory syncytial virus (RSV) (children): CFT;
  (f) Influenza A and B: CFT or hemagglutination inhibition;
  (g) Parainfluenza 1, 2 and 3: CFT;
  (h) Adenovirus: CFT;
  (i) Measles virus: CFT against S & V antigens.

(2) *Opportunist and nosocomial pneumonia* The same tests are used as for acute community-acquired pneumonia, together with the following:

  (a) Cytomegalovirus: CFT, viral culture of urine/blood (detection of early antigenic fluorescent foci (DEAFF) test);
  (b) Varicella zoster virus and herpes simplex: CFT;
  (c) *Aspergillus* spp. precipitins: galactomannan antigen detection;
  (d) *Cryptococcus neoformans*: antigen detection;
  (e) *Mycoplasma pneumoniae*: CFT;
  (f) Epstein–Barr virus: Monospot test, Paul–Bunnell test, specific IgG against viral capsid antigen;
  (g) *Toxoplasma gondii*: enzyme-linked immunosorbent assay (ELISA), dye test;
  (h) HIV 1 and 2: ELISA, immunoblot;
  (i) Human T-cell leukemia virus I (HTLV I): ELISA.

(3) *Tropical and other travel-associated pneumonias*
The same tests are used as for acute community-acquired pneumonia plus the following, according to the country of origin (mostly ELISAs):

(a) *Rickettsia rickettsiae*;
(b) *Coccidioides immitis*;
(c) *Paracoccidioides brasiliensis*;
(d) *Blastomyces dermatitidis*;
(e) *Cryptococcus neoformans*;
(f) *Histoplasma capsulatum*;
(g) *Pseudomonas pseudomallei*;
(h) *Toxoplasma gondii*;
(i) *Strongyloides stercoralis*;
(j) *Schistosoma* spp.;
(k) *Echinococcus granulosus*;
(l) *Paragonimus westermani*;
(m) *Ascaris lumbricoides*;
(n) *Yersinia pestis*.

Pneumococcal antigen can be detected in urine or serum by countercurrent immunoelectrophoresis (CIE) or agglutination tests; in practice, few laboratories perform CIE.

(4) *New methods*   Investigators have developed and investigated a wide variety of laboratory tests for the rapid diagnosis of pneumonia. These tests promise earlier recognition and treatment of infection, and might therefore reduce the morbidity and mortality associated with pneumonia. Examples of tests under evaluation are listed below:

(a) Biotin-labelled probes and polymerase chain reaction (mycobacteria, *Pneumocystis*, respiratory syncytial virus, *Chlamydia* spp., cytomegalovirus, *Pseudomonas pseudomallei*);

(b) An ELISA of urine has been used to detect antigens of *Legionella pneumophila* in urine, and antibodies to *M. tuberculosis* (A5 and A60 and other antigens);

(c) DNA probes for *Nocardia asteroides*;

(d) Adenosine deaminase detection in tuberculous empyema and pneumonias due to other organisms;

(e) Lipoligosaccharide assay for detection of *Haemophilus influenzae* type b.

These tests are of considerable promise though, as yet, without routine practical application in the laboratory.

Tuberculin skin testing can be of some value if positive but does not, of course, exclude mycobacterial infection if negative. Other skin tests, for sarcoidosis and sensitivity to allergens, may help to exclude non-infectious causes of pulmonary disease, if the etiology is uncertain.

Radiological and other pulmonary investigations   In addition to standard radiological investigations such as the posterior–anterior or lateral chest radiograph, the clinician has lately been assisted by dramatic progress in radiological techniques. Computerized tomography, magnetic resonance imaging, radionucleide scans, ventilation-perfusion scans and gas transfer studies are particularly appropriate for identifying non-infective pulmonary pathology which may be difficult to distinguish from an infective process, but may be very helpful in the investigation of lung infections. Computerized tomography (CT) is useful for determining the extent of bronchiectasis, and radionucleide scanning using gallium-67 is an alternative to lung biopsy for detecting infection with *Pneumocystis carinii* in patients with AIDS.

In addition, techniques such as fluoroscopy-guided biopsy can facilitate diagnostic sampling. Bronchography is now rarely required due to the advent of flexible bronchoscopy, but thoracic CT scanning can be modified by injecting contrast media via the bronchoscope. A barium swallow is a valuable investigation to demonstrate esophageal lesions, such as achalasia and gastroesophageal reflux, which may be responsible for pulmonary infection.

Other relevant investigations For the diagnosis of infection there is a wide range of non-specific tests which can assist the clinician. These include:

(1) Peripheral white blood count, blood-film and bone marrow biopsy;

(2) Lung function tests, urea and electrolytes;

(3) Immunoglobulins, C-reactive protein;

(4) Urine studies for cardiovascular disease;

(5) Kveim test, lymph node biopsy;

(6) Avian precipitins;

(7) Lumbar puncture in suspected cryptococcosis or disseminated tuberculosis;

(8) CT head scan in suspected nocardiosis.

Conclusion

Clinicians caring for patients with lower respiratory tract infection now have a wide range of diagnostic tests at their disposal, and an ever-increasing selection of antimicrobials with which to treat them. From these choices, they have a responsibility, in consultation with colleagues in the diagnostic support services, to select the most rational and cost-effective tests for their patients and to interpret the results carefully. We hope that this Atlas will contribute to these objectives.

Routine bronchial infections

Introduction

Infections of the respiratory tract are amongst the most common infections in humans. The majority are caused by viruses (rhinoviruses, influenza and para-influenza) and occur in healthy individuals. Those affected infrequently require medical attention and a specific diagnosis is not obtained. This section concentrates on lower respiratory tract infections in patients with pre-existing lung disease requiring both diagnosis and treatment.

Chronic airways obstruction (synonymous with chronic bronchitis and emphysema) is the most common cause of absenteeism, accounting for 30 million working days lost each year. The majority of illnesses will be due to infection, either viral or bacterial, and infection is responsible for a high proportion of deaths amongst this group. Known risk factors are cigarette smoking, low socioeconomic class, male sex, exposure to atmospheric pollution, repeated childhood respiratory infections and a family history.

Bronchiectasis results in a predisposition to infections due to collections of necrotic material and bronchial secretions in dilated bronchi. It may be caused by infections, usually in childhood, such as pertussis, measles or tuberculosis, and by bronchial obstruction due to inhalation of a foreign body, cystic fibrosis, hypo-gammaglobulinemia and allergic bronchopulmonary aspergillosis. Bronchiectasis is associated with dextro-cardia and sinusitis in Kartagener's syndrome.

Haemophilus influenzae is the most important organism in sustaining inflammation in patients with bronchiectasis. In children with cystic fibrosis, *Staphylococcus aureus* is important, but eventually colonization by *Pseudomonas aeruginosa* occurs. *Pseudomonas (Burkholderia) cepacia* has recently been found to be an important organism in these patients.

This chapter covers routine bacterial infections in patients with chronic airways obstruction and bronchiectasis.

Chronic airways obstruction

Figures 1 and 2 illustrate the case of a 69-year-old lifelong smoker who was admitted with an acute exacerbation of chronic airways obstruction. The anterior–posterior chest radiograph in Figure 1 shows massively hyperinflated lung fields with more than seven anterior ribs visible and a low flat diaphragm. Enlargement of the retrosternal translucent zone (greater than 4 cm) on the lateral radiograph in Figure 2 (measured from the back of the sternum to the anterior aspect of the lower ascending aorta) provides additional radiographic evidence of hyperinflation. An area of consolidation is visible at the left base. Sputum grew *Haemophilus influenzae*, the most common organism to cause infection in this group.

Emphysema

Emphysema is defined as an increase, beyond normal, of air spaces distal to the terminal bronchiole, due to either dilatation or destruction of the walls. Purists would say emphysema is a histological diagnosis but others make the diagnosis on clinical features, lung function and radiographic appearances. The CT scan in Figure 7 shows complete destruction of the lung and formation of emphysematous bullae.

Bronchiectasis

Bronchiectasis, illustrated in Figure 8, is a consequence of infections with bacteria, fungi (e.g. aspergillosis) or viruses, as well as the inherited conditions (e.g. cystic fibrosis and Kartagener's syndrome). Infections cause an inflammatory reaction culminating in lysis of collagen, elastin and often structural proteins of the bronchial wall. Dilatation of the airways inhibits sputum clearance and the warm, moist environment predisposes to infections with anaerobes, *H. influenzae,* streptococci and staphylococci. Later on in the disease, following multiple courses of antibiotics, colonization by *Pseudomonas* spp. occurs; *Pseudomonas aeruginosa* is found in 70–80% of patients with cystic fibrosis.

Bronchograms have now become almost obsolete in the diagnosis of bronchiectasis but may be used as a tool for defining an area of bronchiectasis prior to surgery. A typical bronchogram (see Figure 59) shows a pattern of bronchiectasis with dilatation of segmental bronchi and distal airways of normal caliber. Clubbing of the fingers is associated with bronchiectasis and is illustrated in Figure 9.

Cystic fibrosis

A child presented at 3 years of age with a history of chest infections starting from the first few months of his life. He also had a history of steatorrhea but had reached developmental milestones and was above the third percentile for height and weight. The chest radiograph in Figure 12 shows hyperinflation with bronchial wall thickening and areas of collapse.

The chest radiograph of a 23-year-old patient in Figure 13 shows prominent pulmonary vessels, in the presence of a normal-sized heart, indicative of pulmonary hypertension. The lung fields show typical changes of bronchiectasis with ring shadows and band shadows representing chronic inflammation and thickening of the wall of the bronchioles. Areas of consolidation are seen in the right apex and left midzone. *Pseudomonas aeruginosa* is found in 70–80% of patients with cystic fibrosis, but in this patient *Pseudomonas cepacia* was isolated from the sputum. Patients with cystic fibrosis have either chronic carriage of this organism or a rapid deterioration in their respiratory condition, often followed by death. Recent studies have shown that colonized patients come from the same geographical background with evidence of regular social contact, further substantiating previous work which suggested person-to-person contact.

Fine-cut CT scans (1.5 cm slices) of the thorax demonstrate well the dilated bronchi and fluid levels of patients with bronchiectasis. An example is given in Figure 14.

Pneumonias

Introduction

The word 'pneumonia' has been used to describe illness resulting from inflammation of the lung since Hippocrates in the fourth century BC. A more complete understanding of the disease did not come about until 1814 when Laennec described three stages of consolidation which are still recognized today – engorgement, red hepatization and grey hepatization. Friedlander, in 1884, isolated bacteria from the lungs of fatal cases of pneumonia using staining techniques developed by Gram and Fraenkel. He named the organism 'pneumoniemikrococcus', now known as the pneumococcus.

The discovery of penicillin and improved microbiological identification techniques resulted in a waning interest in pneumonia. However, it then became apparent that there was another group of pneumonias which were not severe and which did not all respond to penicillin. These were called 'atypical pneumonias' and were subsequently found to be caused by organisms such as *Chlamydia psittaci*, *Coxiella burnetii* and *Mycoplasma pneumoniae*. In 1976, a major outbreak of 'Legionnaire's disease' led to the discovery of the organism *Legionella pneumophila* and to further interest in pneumonia as a major cause of morbidity and mortality.

In Britain, one person per 1000 is admitted to hospital with pneumonia each year. The availability of antibiotics has reduced mortality in young adults; however, amongst the elderly mortality is increasing.

Overall, the mortality rate is 5–10% and is influenced by age, being highest in the elderly and young, the organism (*Streptococcus pneumoniae*, *Staphylococcus aureus* and *Klebsiella*), pre-existing lung disease, and underlying immunosuppression.

Pneumonia can conveniently be classified according to the circumstances in which it was acquired, and can be divided into community-acquired pneumonia and hospital-acquired pneumonia. The majority of cases of community-acquired pneumonia are primary infections but secondary bacterial infection is common in outbreaks of influenza or in chronic airways obstruction. Hospital-acquired pneumonia usually occurs in patients with impaired immunity or pre-existing disease. Pneumonia in AIDS patients is of increasing importance and is discussed in a later section.

Community-acquired pneumonia is most often caused by viruses, *Streptococcus pneumoniae*, *Mycoplasma pneumoniae*, and then less commonly by *Chlamydia pneumoniae*, *Haemophilus influenzae* and *Staphylococcus aureus*. *H. influenzae* usually affects those with lung disease but rarely affects healthy young adults. Gram-negative cocci such as *Neisseria meningitidis* and *Moraxella catarrhalis* infrequently cause pneumonia.

The increase in numbers of patients profoundly immunosuppressed following organ transplantation or chemotherapy has resulted in a continued rise in hospital-acquired pneumonia. Pneumococci, *Staphylococcus aureus*, coliforms or *Pseudomonas* sp. are common causes of bacterial infections in postoperative patients in intensive care, and anaerobes are important pathogens in patients with aspiration pneumonia. Organisms such as cytomegalovirus, *Pneumocystis carinii*, *Nocardia* and *Aspergillus* spp. are important causes of infection in the compromised host.

This section covers community- and hospital-acquired pneumonia, starting with the more common organisms, although other examples may be found elsewhere in the Atlas. Lung abscesses and pleuropulmonary diseases are also included here.

Community-acquired pneumonias

Pneumococcal pneumonia
Figures 19 and 20 illustrate the case of a 41-year-old smoker who 3 weeks prior to admission had a 'flu-like illness. She presented with right-sided chest and abdominal pain, and a cough productive of blood-stained sputum. Clinically, she had signs of right lower and middle lobe pneumonia. Her condition deteriorated rapidly and within 12 h of admission she required intubation, mechanical ventilation and inotropic support. Her chest radiographs (Figures 19 and 20) show right middle and lower lobar consolidation with a right-sided pleural effusion. Blood cultures grew *Streptococcus pneumoniae* (Figure 21).

Staphylococcal pneumonia
Staphylococcus aureus is responsible for less than 5% of all cases of pneumonia but is important due to its high morbidity. In children it often follows a mild viral respiratory illness and is characterized by a rapid deterioration in the child's clinical condition; in adults it may follow influenza virus infection.

The chest radiograph of a small child (Figure 27) shows widespread bilateral infiltrates with pneumatocele

formation characteristic of this organism. Volume loss, cavitation and pleural effusion or empyema are common features.

Moraxella catarrhalis *pneumonia*
Moraxella catarrhalis is an unusual cause of pneumonia and normally occurs in patients who are immuno-compromised or who have chronic lung disease. The chest radiograph in Figure 30 shows left lower lobe consolidation and a left pleural effusion. The patient failed to respond to ampicillin and erythromycin but responded to a cephalosporin with both clinical and radiographic resolution. *Moraxella catarrhalis* was isolated from his sputum.

Mycoplasma pneumoniae *pneumonia*
The most common cause of atypical community-acquired pneumonia is infection with *Mycoplasma pneumoniae*. Mild epidemics are seen every 4 years. Symptoms of upper respiratory tract and bronchial infections are common and pneumonia occurs in only 25% of cases. Non-respiratory symptoms are numerous.

A fine reticular pattern (Figures 31–33), which may be unilateral or bilateral, and which later may progress to patchy consolidation, often distinguishes mycoplasma pneumonia from other bacterial pneumonias. Lower lobe involvement is usually confined to children.

Histoplasmosis
Histoplasmosis is a fungal infection caused by *Histoplasma capsulatum* and is commonly seen in Canada and North America, particularly on the Eastern side. Most cases are asymptomatic and are diagnosed by skin tests and evidence of calcified foci on a chest radiograph. Occasional epidemics of symptomatic infections are reported.

The chest radiograph in Figure 36 of an asymptomatic patient depicts calcified foci in the lungs and in lymph nodes in the hila and mediastinum. The rounded granulomas are known as histoplasmomas and have a fibrous capsule consisting of concentric laminations. Calcification of these laminations is specific for histoplasmosis.

Chlamydia psittaci *pneumonia*

Chlamydia psittaci is responsible for only 2–5% of adult community-acquired pneumonias. Figure 38 shows the case of a 49-year-old-lady who presented with a 3-day history of an upper respiratory tract infection, headache, photophobia and a dry cough. She denied contact with birds. She was pyrexial with a macular rash on her back ('Horden's spots') and the chest radiograph shows segmental consolidation in the lateral segment of the right lower lobe. She responded to oral erythromycin. A greater than four-fold increase in complement-fixing antibodies to *Chlamydia psittaci* was measured in her serum.

Chlamydia psittaci is endemic in avian species including psittacine birds, canaries, finches, pigeons and poultry. Birds are frequently asymptomatic carriers but excretion of the organism is associated with transport, illness and overcrowding.

Chlamydia trachomatis *pneumonia*

This organism usually produces lower respiratory tract infections in the first weeks of life. The full-term neonate in Figure 39 was 2 weeks of age when he developed respiratory distress. Serology revealed *Chlamydia trachomatis* as the causative organism. The radiographic appearances are variable and indistinguishable from those produced by viruses or pertussis.

Coxiella burnetii *or Q fever*

Q fever is characterized by an abrupt onset of fever, headache, general malaise and weakness. The chest radiograph in Figure 42 shows an area of consolidation which is radiologically indistinguishable from other atypical pneumonias. A complete recovery was made

following a course of tetracycline. A proportion of patients go on to develop hepatitis or endocarditis. The diagnosis was confirmed by a four-fold increase in specific antibodies to *Coxiella burnetii*.

Respiratory syncytial virus

Respiratory syncytial virus causes bronchiolitis and pneumonia and represents the most common lower respiratory tract infection in young children, typically less than 1 year old.

The chest radiographs in Figure 43 show diffuse air trapping, manifest by hyperinflation and low flat diaphragms. Peribronchial thickening produces ring shadows or parallel linear shadows. When the infection spreads to the lung causing pneumonia, areas of atelectasis are also seen. Patients recovering from viral pneumonia may have radiographic abnormalities for weeks but complete resolution usually occurs.

Influenza pneumonia

Pneumonia as a complication of influenza virus infection can be a primary viral or secondary bacterial infection. Figure 47 illustrates the case of an elderly gentleman in a geriatric ward where an influenza outbreak occurred over the winter months. He had a 2-day 'flu-like illness followed by a non-productive cough and nasal discharge. His chest radiograph shows right lower zone consolidation. In this case no bacterial pathogens were found in the sputum, the white cell count was normal and the patient failed to respond to antibiotics. Influenza virus was isolated from nasal swabs and nasopharyngeal aspirate, and a serological diagnosis was made retrospectively. Influenza A is the most common type causing pneumonia in adults. In epidemics the prevalence is increased; only a minority of patients develop pneumonic shadowing.

Bordetella pertussis *pneumonia*

Figure 48 shows the chest radiograph of a 2-year-old non-immunized child requiring mechanical ventilation for *Bordetella pertussis* pneumonia. The illness started with coryzal symptoms and developed within 2 weeks into a classical paroxysmal cough with an inspiratory whoop, terminating in vomiting. Prior to ventilation the child had an anoxic fit. The chest radiograph shows bronchial wall thickening, consolidation with areas of atelectasis, and an endotracheal tube. Pharyngeal aspirate and swabs did not culture the organism but paired antibody titers confirmed the diagnosis.

Varicella zoster viral pneumonia

Figure 50 illustrates the case of a 44-year-old Sri Lankan man who presented with acute severe pneumonia requiring mechanical ventilation. He had a history of exposure to chickenpox and had developed a rash one week earlier. He developed a cough with shortness of breath 3 days prior to admission. Following intubation, a bronchoscopy was performed and vesicles were seen throughout the airways. He failed to respond to treatment and died. Varicella zoster virus is unusual as it causes pneumonia more frequently in adults than in children and the case illustrated here demonstrates the potential seriousness of the disease.

Young adults with this disease often have predisposing risk factors such as lymphoma, pregnancy or immunosuppressive therapy. The 46-year-old otherwise healthy adult shown in Figure 51 was being contact-traced for tuberculosis. She had a history of recent chickenpox but had no respiratory symptoms. Previous chest radiographs were normal but this chest radiograph shows multiple small nodules in both lungs up to 7 mm in diameter and characteristic of chickenpox. Nodules are classically 5–10 mm in diameter and either come and go or become confluent (see Figure 50). They can persist for months and in 2% of cases they calcify, as illustrated in Figure 56 which shows a routine chest radiograph of a medical student, on arrival at Medical School, who was not aware of a history of chickenpox. Calcification primarily affects the mid to lower zone and the nodules are usually less than 3 mm in diameter.

Measles (giant cell) pneumonia

In Figure 55, a 28-year-old gardener presented with a 4-day history of an unproductive cough following a 'flu-like illness. She went on to develop a productive cough and fever. On examination, she had Koplik spots and a truncal macular rash. The chest radiograph shows widespread primary viral pneumonia with extensive bilateral confluent shadowing and a right pleural effusion. The left pulmonary artery is prominent as a consequence of an atrial septal defect repair at the age of 18 years.

Allergic bronchopulmonary aspergillosis

Allergic bronchopulmonary aspergillosis is an immunological reaction to *Aspergillus fumigatus* spores, so is not truly a lung infection. It usually presents in asthmatic subjects with expectoration of brown plugs, an eosinophilia and transient lung infiltrates. The condition is confirmed by circulating precipitins and positive immediate and/or late skin prick reactions to *A. fumigatus*. A chest radiograph (Figure 56) in the acute phase may be normal or reveal bilateral airspace shadowing. Between attacks the chest radiograph may return to normal (Figure 57), but often in the subacute phase reticulonodular shadowing is apparent (Figure 58). Repeated attacks result in pulmonary fibrosis and bronchiectasis.

Coccidioides immitis pneumonia

Coccidioides immitis is a fungus which grows in the soil in arid and semi-desert conditions. The main endemic areas are southwestern USA, and arid zones in Guatemala, Honduras, Columbia, Argentina and Uruguay.

The majority of infections are subclinical and 80–90% of people living in an endemic area may develop positive skin tests without overt disease. Acute respiratory infection (Valley fever), however, is characterized by fever, malaise and cough. Arthralgia and toxic erythema, erythema nodosum or erythema multiforme are also commonly associated.

The chest radiographic appearances range from patchy consolidation, usually of lower lobes, associated with a pleural effusion, to hilar or mediastinal lymph node enlargement. The chest radiograph shown in Figure 59 shows a left mid-zone infiltrate associated with left hilar lymphadenopathy. The computed tomographic scan (Figure 60) shows the lesion to be abutting on the pleura and to contain an area of necrosis. Large left hilar nodes are visible.

Hospital-acquired pneumonias

Klebsiella pneumonia
Typical features of klebsiella pneumonia are consolidation, particularly of the right upper lobe, with cavitation and a pleural effusion. A 30-year-old lady required liver transplantation following a paracetamol overdose. Her recovery was complicated by recurrent chest infections and a tracheostomy was required. Six weeks post-transplantation, she developed a left subpulmonary effusion; cultures of bronchial washings and pleural fluid yielded a multiply antibiotic-resistant Klebsiella pneumoniae (Figures 61 and 62). An outbreak of klebsiella infection subsequently occurred on the ward.

Staphylococcus epidermidis pneumonia
Figure 63 illustrates the case of a premature neonate who was one of a set of twins. He developed respiratory distress syndrome and required ventilation. The chest radiograph shows a ground-glass appearance consistent with the diagnosis and right upper zone consolidation. Repeated blood cultures grew Staphylococcus epidermidis which was considered to be the cause of the pneumonia. Caution must be taken in attributing this organism to the cause of pneumonia in neonatal units and a careful search must be made for other organisms.

Group B streptococcus
A 30-week-old preterm infant developed respiratory distress within hours of birth. The chest radiograph in Figure 66 demonstrates confluent opacification of the lungs with air bronchograms and the loss of all mediastinal and diaphragmatic borders. The neonate was found to be neutropenic and Group B streptococcus was grown from blood cultures of mother and neonate. The changes of congenital pneumonia are indistinguishable from those of neonatal respiratory distress syndrome.

Legionella pneumonia
The series of chest radiographs in Figures 69–71 shows consolidation in the right lower lobe in a ventilated patient (Figure 69), spread to involve both lung fields (Figure 70) (note the Swan–Ganz catheter in place) and marked improvement in the consolidation (Figure 71). The most typical radiological pattern is unilateral and peripheral lower zone consolidation with rapid progression commonly involving other lobes on the same or opposite side. Pleural effusion occurs in up to 50% of patients but is not usually a dominant feature. Resolution is often slow and may be interrupted by new areas of consolidation. This 61-year-old renal transplant patient had severe legionella pneumonia. Patients at risk of developing this type of pneumonia are elderly smokers, alcoholics, diabetics and the immunosuppressed. The diagnosis was confirmed by L. pneumophila titers and the source was found to be the water supply to the ward.

Nocardia
Nocardia rarely causes severe infection other than in the immunosuppressed. The renal transplant patient in Figure 74 had been well for 5 years when she presented with a fever. A chest radiograph shows a solitary lesion in the right lower zone with some patchy consolidation in the right upper zone. Culture of material obtained from fine needle aspiration grew Nocardia asteroides, the most common Nocardia spp. to cause pulmonary infection. Pleural involvement and

empyema formation are common. Cavitating lesions may also be seen.

Cytomegalovirus pneumonitis

Figures 78 and 79 illustrate the case of a 42-year-old lady who had an orthotopic liver transplant for primary biliary cirrhosis. Postoperatively, she developed pneumonia and a chest radiograph taken at this time (Figure 78) shows consolidation of the right middle lobe. Her condition deteriorated over the next 2 weeks and she required mechanical ventilation. Her chest radiograph (Figure 79) shows extensive bilateral infiltrates, although bronchoalveolar lavage was negative for organisms. The cytomegalovirus complement fixation test prior to transplant was negative in the patient and donor, but a liver biopsy showed cytomegalovirus inclusion bodies and, despite empirical treatment for cytomegalovirus, the patient died. The cytomegalovirus complement fixation test (IgM) was positive at this stage and infection was presumed to have come from transfused blood.

Cytomegalovirus pneumonitis is seen in immunosuppressed patients and often co-pathogens like bacteria and Pneumocystis carinii are also isolated.

Aspergillus spp. pneumonia

Aspergillus spp. may become invasive in the immunocompromised host and is an important cause of pneumonia in these patients. A 64-year-old man was receiving chemotherapy for acute transformation of chronic myeloid leukemia. The chest radiograph in Figure 82 shows typical non-specific patchy consolidation with multiple large nodules which may, in time, cavitate.

The diagnosis was made from bronchoscopic washings which revealed fungal hyphae on direct microscopy; Aspergillus fumigatus was grown after 3 days' culture on Sabouraud's agar.

During follow-up for a mitral valve replacement, the 53-year-old lady shown in Figure 83 had a cough productive of green sputum, intermittent fevers and weight loss. Twelve years earlier she had received conventional antituberculous agents for pulmonary tuberculosis. The chest radiograph shows bilateral apical fibrosis with a cavitating mass on the right. Sputum examination was repeatedly negative for acid-alcohol-fast bacilli but culture grew Aspergillus fumigatus. Serum precipitins for Aspergillus spp. were positive, although the eosinophil count was normal.

Pulmonary mycetomas are formed by the colonization of a cavity secondary to a chronic inflammatory process such as tuberculosis, sarcoidosis, or histoplasmosis. Mycetomas have also been recognized in emphysematous bullae, congenital lung cysts and cavitating bronchial carcinomas.

Strongyloides hyperinfection

A 27-year-old Ghanaian man was receiving chemotherapy for adult T-cell leukemia lymphoma associated with human T cell lymphotrophic virus type I (HTLV I). He developed fever, meningism, abdominal pain and distension, and his radiograph (Figure 87) showed extensive reticulonodular shadowing. Strongyloides larvae were seen in feces, sputum and duodenal aspirate. Treatment with thiabendazole resulted in clearance of strongyloides larvae within 10 days, and radiological improvement a few weeks later.

Lung abscesses and other infections

Lung abscess is an infection resulting in suppurative inflammation, necrosis and cavitation of the lung. This may result from aspiration, bronchial obstruction, septicemia, direct spread from hepatic or subphrenic abscesses or as a complication of a pneumonia, particularly Klebsiella spp. or Staphylococcus aureus (see Figure 27).

Staphylococcal abscess

Figures 89 and 90 show the case of a 45-year-old woman who presented postoperatively with a 3-week history of persistent cough productive of purulent sputum and fevers. The chest radiograph revealed a large abscess in the right upper lobe and *Staphylococcus aureus* was cultured from the pus. Abscesses usually result from aspiration after an episode of altered consciousness, in this case, surgery. Consolidation is either uni- or multifocal and is most commonly seen in posterior upper, apical lower or posterobasal segments of the right lung.

Streptococcus milleri *abscess*

The patient shown in Figure 91 had a history of diarrhea and protracted vomiting. His chest radiograph showed basal consolidation. Computerized tomography demonstrates cavitation of the consolidation within the lung parenchyma. Blood cultures and pus extracted from the patient's right maxillary sinus grew *Streptococcus milleri*. Liver biopsy showed no evidence of abscesses, lymphoma or granuloma and no underlying cause of the infection was found.

Streptococcus milleri (recently renamed *Strep. intermedius*) is the most common organism, aerobic or anaerobic, to be found in lung abscesses. Other common pathogenic aerobic organisms causing lung abscesses are *Streptococcus pneumoniae*, *Staphylococcus aureus*, *Klebsiella* spp. and *Haemophilus influenzae*.

Aspiration pneumonia

Abscesses are present in both lung fields of the patient shown in Figure 93. Aspiration from the oropharynx is the most common cause of lung abscesses. Predisposing factors are:-

(1) Impaired consciousness, such as caused by alcohol/drug abuse, or anesthesia;

(2) Lower cranial nerve lesions, for example, infective polyneuritis;

(3) Weakness of the musculature of the pharynx, larynx and esophagus, for example from muscular dystrophy;

(4) Pharyngeal pouch;

(5) Laryngeal tumor;

(6) Esophageal stricture, for example caused by carcinoma, achalasia.

Hydatid cyst

The 60-year-old male from the Middle East shown in Figure 96 presented with a pyrexial illness and cough. The chest radiograph shows a rounded area of consolidation in the right lower zone and some air is seen within the lesion. The edges are ill defined and this represents a collapsed hydatid cyst. The right lower lobe is the commonest site.

The 34-year-old Turkish man shown in Figure 97 presented with cough, hemoptysis, fever and weight loss. A Mantoux test was positive and the chest radiograph findings were consistent with tuberculosis. The sputum was positive for acid-alcohol-fast bacilli. The large lobulated cyst on the right was an incidental finding. Immunoelectrophoresis for antibodies to *Echinococcus granulosus* confirmed the diagnosis.

A magnetic resonance imaging scan of the patient in Figure 98 shows a well-defined fluid-filled cyst on a T1 weighted image. The membranes are not visible and no daughter cysts are seen. The consolidation on the left has now resolved following antituberculous therapy.

Pleuropulmonary infection

Empyema is a purulent pleural effusion which normally follows a pulmonary infection – pneumonia, lung abscess or bronchiectasis. It may occur following septicemia, thoracic surgery or a penetrating chest wound or from transdiaphragmatic spread from subphrenic or hepatic abscesses.

Infection within the pleural space results in an inflammatory exudate, the production of fibrinous adhesions, which may lead to loculation and eventually deposition of fibrin, and progressive fibrosis. Bronchopulmonary fistulae may develop during the inflammatory phase. Fibrosis leads to a restrictive defect and chest wall deformity. Early intercostal drainage and, when indicated, decortication of the pleura, along with appropriate antibiotic therapy, will prevent permanent sequelae.

Empyema

A 70-year-old man with pre-existing lung disease presented with a productive cough and fever. His chest radiograph (Figure 100) demonstrates a large right-sided pleural effusion with hyperinflation and bullae in the right upper zone. Bronchiectasis is prominent in the left lower zone. Aspiration of the fluid revealed sterile purulent material. CT scans of the thorax of the same patient (Figure 101) demonstrate the volume of the empyema and pre-existing lung damage.

Actinomycosis

A 30-year-old woman presented with a 3-week history of a mild febrile illness and a dry cough. The chest radiograph in Figure 104 shows consolidation of the right upper lobe and part of the lower lobe with an air bronchogram. Periosteal reaction is demonstrated along the lower border of the posterior ends of the right ribs indicating rib involvement (see arrow). *Actinomyces israelii* was found in the sputum. Cervical disc involvement at the level of C6–7 led to meningitis and the death of the patient.

Schistosomiasis

The 45-year-old Indian shown in Figure 106 had lived in Kenya for 16 years. He presented in the UK with ankle swelling and breathlessness. On examination, he had a raised jugular venous pressure with a loud pulmonic sound and bilateral coarse basal crackles. His chest radiograph confirms the diagnosis of pulmonary hypertension with prominent pulmonary vessels. Interstitial shadowing is seen throughout the lung fields. The diagnosis was confirmed by open lung biopsy which demonstrated interstitial fibrosis, thickened alveolar walls, hypertensive vessel changes and old occluded and recanalized blood vessels. Liver biopsy confirmed the diagnosis.

Pulmonary hypertension sometimes results from embolization of the eggs in very severe cases, but more often from those with large portal-systemic circulations resulting from hepatosplenic schistosomiasis. This allows a large number of eggs to bypass the liver and become trapped in capillary beds, leading to arteritis and pulmonary hypertension.

Mycobacterium tuberculosis

Introduction

In Victorian England one person in five died from tuberculosis. The identification of *Mycobacterium tuberculosis* as the causative organism by Koch in 1882 was the first major step in our understanding of the condition, and, although public health measures, introduced on the basis of this knowledge, helped to some extent to control the spread of the condition, it was not until the 1940s that immunization schemes and effective antituberculous drugs became available. Since then there has been a steep decline in the incidence and prevalence of the condition in 'developed' countries.

It has, however, remained a formidable problem in the Third World. Furthermore, the decline in the Western world has been halted, and in some countries reverted to an increase, by the advent of AIDS-related tuberculosis. This problem is of an order of magnitude greater in sub-Saharan Africa where, in some countries, 50–60% of newly diagnosed cases of tuberculosis are found to be HIV positive.

Primary pulmonary tuberculosis is usually an airborne infection from a sputum-positive patient and results, in most otherwise healthy people, in a small lesion in the lungs. This heals, and leads to a substantial degree of subsequent immunity. Post-primary infection is either from reinfection, or reactivation of persistent viable organisms. Risk factors for the disease include diabetes mellitus, malnutrition, social deprivation, alcoholism and immunosuppression.

Treatment with appropriate antituberculous drugs is highly effective, and public health programs for prevention of spread have also played an important part in the decline of the disease. However, as the world-wide incidence of AIDS increases and the Third-World social conditions continue to be a problem, tuberculosis has re-acquired its status as an infection of major significance.

Post-primary infection from *Mycobacterium tuberculosis*

Figures 108 and 109 illustrate the case of a 33-year-old Irish laborer who presented with cough, breathlessness and weight loss over 3 months. In the preceding 3 weeks he had developed night sweats and hemoptysis. The chest radiograph in Figure 108 shows cavitating left upper zone shadowing with evidence of collapse, and a shift of the trachea and mediastinum to the left. After 9 months of antituberculous treatment and corticosteroids, he had persistent upper zone shadowing indicative of fibrosis (Figure 109).

Diffuse pneumonia

The chest radiograph in Figure 110 shows diffuse nodular shadowing throughout both lung fields with cavitation and collapse of the right upper lobe. These nodules are consistent with consolidation following bronchogenic spread from the right upper lobe.

Hilar lymphadenopathy

The chest radiograph in Figure 111 is from a 32-year-old Indian lady who presented with fever, general malaise and a non-productive cough. Two of her children had chest radiographs suggestive of tuberculosis. She had a good response clinically to antituberculous agents but radiological appearances did not improve. A mediastinoscopy and biopsy confirmed infection with *Mycobacterium tuberculosis*.

Patients from the Indian subcontinent often have mediastinal node involvement in post-primary disease.

Miliary shadowing

Magnification of the chest radiograph in Figure 112 demonstrates the 'millet seeds' of miliary shadowing which results from hematogenous spread following primary infection. The younger the age at which primary infection occurs, the higher the incidence of miliary tuberculosis. The chest radiograph illustrated is of a 25-year-old Indian man returning from the Indian subcontinent.

Tuberculous empyema

Figures 113 and 114 show the case of a 28-year-old bus conductor who presented with a pyrexial illness and weight loss. His chest radiograph (Figure 113) shows a left pleural effusion. Aspiration was not possible on the ward and the patient underwent a mini-thoracotomy and insertion of a chest drain. The pleural aspirate was initially sterile but, after 6 weeks, *Mycobacterium tuberculosis* was grown. Complete recovery resulted from a full course of antituberculous therapy. The CT scan of the thorax (Figure 114) reveals the empyema with no underlying pathology. Tuberculous empyema carries a poorer prognosis than primary tuberculosis and can lead to pleural thickening and calcification, resulting in a restrictive lung defect.

Old tuberculous empyema

The chest radiograph in Figure 115 demonstrates marked bilateral pleural calcification following a tuberculous empyema in the days prior to treatment with early drainage and corticosteroids. Tuberculous lesions show a marked tendency to calcification, a radiological hallmark of tuberculous disease.

The acquired immune deficiency syndrome

Introduction

The pandemic of HIV infection has had an incalculable effect on global health care, both in industrialized and developing countries. By the end of the century, an estimated 20–30 million people will be infected. The respiratory tract is, of course, a major site of infection in AIDS, and several diseases (such as infection with *Pneumocystis carinii* and *Mycobacterium avium* complex) are included as AIDS-defining illnesses. Ironically, the opportunist infections in AIDS patients have provided much useful information on the role of cell-mediated and other host defence mechanisms in the respiratory tract.

Patients with severe lower respiratory tract infection must be questioned carefully to determine if there is any history of risk behavior for HIV infection. Many clinicians will recall incidents, particularly in the early 1980s, when underlying HIV infection was considered only after patients were found to be infected with unusual opportunist pathogens, and after the patient had deteriorated considerably while receiving conventional antibiotic therapy. As well as direct questioning about risk behavior for HIV, indirect evidence for AIDS may be gathered from systematic questioning and clinical examination. This evidence consists of:

(1) Intravenous drug injection sites;

(2) Evidence of protracted weight loss and general malaise in a previously healthy individual;

(3) Protracted concurrent diarrheal disease;

(4) Oropharyngeal candidiasis;

(5) Kaposi's sarcoma manifesting as skin and mucous membrane lesions.

The diagnostic approach to pneumonia in the patient with known or suspected HIV infection is, of necessity, notably different from that in patients without HIV. The clinician must take into account the following important factors:

(1) Duration of AIDS, and CD4 counts. Infections due to *Mycobacterium avium* complex tend to appear at later stages of the illness with low CD4 counts, whereas pneumocystis pneumonia is a common presenting illness;

(2) Occurrence of past episodes of pneumonia and concurrent antimicrobial prophylaxis or treatment for pneumocystis, fungi, mycobacteria, etc.;

(3) Geographical setting, e.g. higher risk of histoplasma, coccidioides in some localities;

(4) Risk of concurrent respiratory pathogens and multiply-resistant mycobacteria.

Because of the wide range of pathogens that may be encountered in these patients, every effort should be made to obtain a specific diagnosis by bronchoalveolar lavage, biopsy, sputum induction and serological tests.

However, it should be noted that patients with typical features of infection with organisms such as *Pneumocystis carinii* are often given empirical therapy, and invasive procedures are performed only if the patient does not respond.

Pneumocystis carinii is the most common opportunistic infection in patients with AIDS in Europe and North America. In the US, 64% of AIDS patients present with *Pneumocystis carinii* pneumonia as their first infection and 80% of AIDS patients acquire *Pneumocystis carinii* at some time during the course of their disease. Almost a third of those infected will have a co-existing pathogen. These include, in decreasing order of frequency, cytomegalovirus, *Mycobacterium avium* complex, *Mycobacterium tuberculosis*, *Legionella* and *Cryptococcus*. Cytomegalovirus is commonly found in the body fluids and tissues of patients with AIDS but rarely causes pulmonary disease. This is in stark contrast to the life-threatening pneumonitis with which cytomegalovirus is associated in patients who are immunocompromised for other reasons, e.g. organ transplantation (p. 24), taking immunosuppressive agents.

Other primary infections in AIDS patients are caused by *Mycobacterium avium* complex, *Cryptococcus*, pyogenic bacteria, *Legionella*, fungi and *M. tuberculosis*. Herpes simplex virus and *Toxoplasma gondii* rarely infect the lung in AIDS patients. Tuberculosis tends to occur earlier than *Pneumocystis carinii* pneumonia in the natural history of HIV infection, and in a considerable number of patients the disease is extrapulmonary. Infection with 'atypical' mycobacteria such as *Mycobacterium avium* complex occurs later in the course of the disease at a stage when treatment may not be effective.

Infection with 'conventional' bacteria is common in patients with HIV infection because of the reduced antibody response and the specific defect of cell-mediated immunity. For this reason, capsulate bacteria such as *Streptococcus pneumoniae* and *Haemophilus influenzae* are a particular problem. Pulmonary infections due to enterobacteria (coliforms) or *Staphylococcus aureus* may be seen late in the course of the illness.

Some of the infections seen in AIDS patients are common in non-AIDS patients and the reader is referred to other sections.

Pneumococcal infection

Figure 120 is a chest radiograph of a 3-year-old Afro-Carribean child who was known to have AIDS following the diagnosis of tuberculosis 1 year earlier. She suffered repeated pneumococcal chest infections responsive to antibiotics. The HIV status of the mother was not established. The chest radiograph shows consolidation in the left mid-zone with right hilar lymphadenopathy. Blood cultures grew *Streptococcus pneumoniae*.

Pneumocystis carinii pneumonia

The chest radiograph in Figure 121 is from a 25-year-old man who presented with a dry cough and breathlessness. Chest examination was normal. Oxygen saturation was normal at rest but desaturated on exercise. An HIV test was positive and lymphocyte subset examination revealed a CD4 count less than 25 cells per μl. Grocott's silver staining of a histological specimen obtained by a transbronchial biopsy revealed *Pneumocystis carinii*.

Of all patients with *Pneumocystis carinii* pneumonia, 4–14% have a normal chest radiograph on presentation. *Pneumocystis carinii* pneumonia can cause localized shadowing but classically causes a bilateral perihilar haze indistinct from pulmonary edema. When the whole lung is involved, there is sparing of the periphery. Pneumothorax is a recognized complication of both the disease and transbronchial biopsy.

Figure 122 is a CT scan of a 38-year-old business man, who had travelled extensively in Africa, and who presented with cough and shortness of breath.

Examination of his chest was normal but the patient was cyanosed and arterial pO_2 was measured at 4 kPa. The CT scan shows marked interstitial change within the lung parenchyma. Immunocytological examination of bronchial washings demonstrated the presence of *Pneumocystis carinii*.

Bilateral apical cavitation is seen in the patient in Figure 123 with *Pneumocystis carinii* pneumonia and is a recognized variant. Histology of these cysts has shown them to contain alveolar exudate and *Pneumocystis carinii*.

The AIDS patient in Figure 124 was diagnosed as having both *Pneumocystis carinii* pneumonia and pulmonary tuberculosis on transbronchial biopsy. In the immunocompromised host, it is not uncommon for such pathogens to co-exist.

Mycobacterium tuberculosis pneumonia

The 25-year-old Ugandan woman in Figure 126 presented with symptoms and signs typical of *Mycobacterium tuberculosis* infection. She failed to respond to first-line antituberculous agents and her white cell count was found to be low. An HIV test was found to be positive.

The chest radiograph in Figure 126 shows right upper zone consolidation with hilar lymphadenopathy typical of tuberculosis, with elevation of the right hemi-diaphragm indicative of underlying fibrosis.

Mycobacterium tuberculosis presents early in the natural history of HIV infection. This is thought to be due to the fact that the pathogenicity of the organism is greater than that of organisms like *Pneumocystis carinii* which cause infection early on. Direct and indirect epidemiological data indicate that the HIV virus has a dominant role in the resurgence of tuberculosis in the US, but in the UK, where the incidence of tuberculosis is also rising, this has not been the case.

Mycobacterium avium complex

Figure 127 is of an AIDS patient who presented with weight loss, increasing debility and shortness of breath late on in the course of his disease. He had profound diarrhea and *Mycobacterium avium* complex was isolated from blood cultures and feces.

Disseminated infection with *Mycobacterium avium* complex is seen in 10–20% of AIDS patients in life and 50% of patients at autopsy. Since the 1950s, it has been recognized as an uncommon cause of pneumonia in immunocompetent patients with lung disease.

Mycobacterium kansasii

The HIV-positive patient shown in Figure 130 grew *Mycobacterium kansasii* from culture of sputum. His chest radiograph shows bilateral cavitating apical shadowing. The radiographic appearances of small thin-walled cavitating masses are indistinguishable from post-primary tuberculosis. However, local pleural thickening with little surrounding parenchymal change is suggestive of an atypical mycobacterium.

Mycobacterium malmoensii

A 27-year-old AIDS patient presented with a productive cough and the chest radiograph in Figure 132 shows a cavitating mass in the left mid-zone, with surrounding parenchymal change but no node involvement. Bronchoscopy was normal but bronchoalveolar lavage was positive for acid-alcohol-fast bacilli. Cultures grew *Mycobacterium malmoensii*.

Coccidioides immitis

Infection by *Coccidioides immitis* is normally asymptomatic in endemic areas although it can cause an acute pulmonary infection (see Figure 59). In immuno-suppressed patients, it may become disseminated to include lung (Figure 135), skin, bone, meninges, and joints. Smears, cultures and serology are all helpful in the diagnosis and monitoring of the course of the infection.

Enlargement of the right lung field of the chest radiograph shown in Figure 135 shows diffuse nodular infiltrates involving the entire lung field. This patient was known to be HIV-positive.

Lymphoid interstitial pneumonia

Figure 137 shows the case of a 2-year-old child whose mother was known to be HIV-positive and who presented with bilateral parotitis and pyrexia. The chest radiograph shows bilateral interstitial disease and hilar lymphadenopathy consistent with the diagnosis of lymphoid interstitial pneumonitis.

Lymphoid interstitial pneumonitis is a condition associated with hypergammaglobulinemia. Histological sections show alveolar septa distended with masses of mature lymphocytes. Children with AIDS characteristically have large numbers of non-functioning CD4 cells and hypergammaglobulinemia, and have a predisposition to lymphoid interstitial pneumonitis. Recently, it has been suggested that this condition is associated with the Epstein–Barr virus.

Section 2   Lung Infections Illustrated

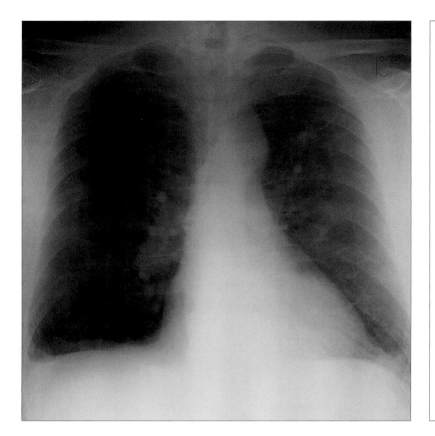

Figure 1 Anteroposterior chest radiograph of chronic airways obstruction in a patient with chronic bronchitis

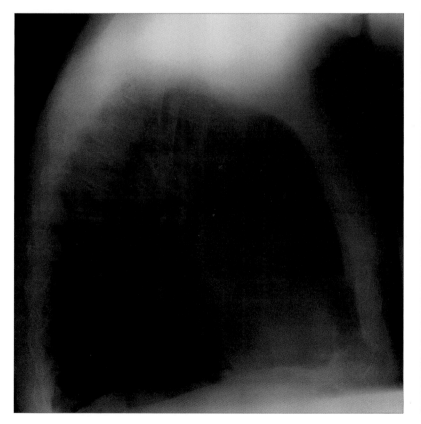

Figure 2 Lateral chest radiograph of chronic airways obstruction in a patient with chronic bronchitis

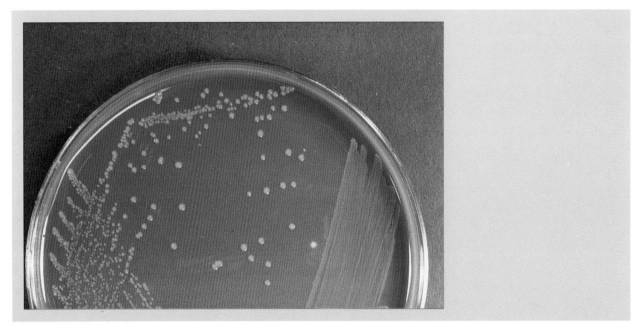

Figure 3 Chocolate blood agar growing *Haemophilus influenzae*. 'Chocolate' blood agar contains heated blood and has high levels of X and V factors, which *Haemophilus influenzae* requires for growth. It is particularly useful for culture of haemophili and other respiratory pathogens such as *Streptococcus pneumoniae*. The agar surface is inoculated with a sample of respiratory tract secretions and is then incubated for 18–24 h in 10% CO_2 at 37°C. *H. influenzae* is identified by its dependence on X and V factors. Both *H. influenzae* and *Streptococcus pneumoniae* may be carried in the respiratory tract, particularly in patients with chronic obstructive airways disease, so their presence does not necessarily indicate disease

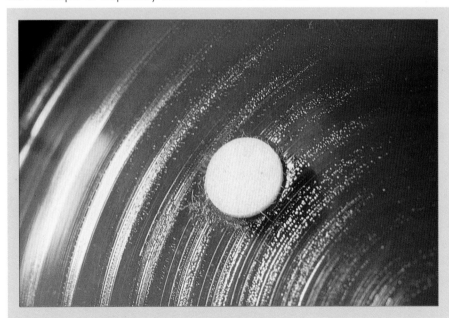

Figure 4 X and V disc for the identification of *Haemophilus* spp. Haemophili are 'blood-loving' (hence the name). *Haemophilus influenzae* is dependent for growth on both hematin (X factor) and NAD or NADP (V factor). This dependence can be used to identify the organism in the laboratory. On nutrient agar, which does not contain blood or serum (so containing neither X nor V), *H. influenzae* only grows around the disc that contains both X and V factors. *H. parainfluenzae*, which is also found in the respiratory tract but rarely causes disease, is dependent on V factor only

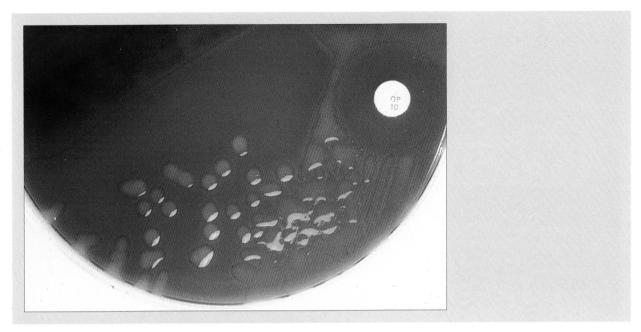

Figure 5 *Streptococcus pneumoniae* on blood agar. The colonies are surrounded by a green halo because *Streptococcus pneumoniae* causes partial hemolysis of the blood agar (α-hemolysis). Capsulate pneumococci may be mucoid, like this one, or they may have 'draughtsman'-shaped colonies, with a central depression in the colony which is a result of autolysis

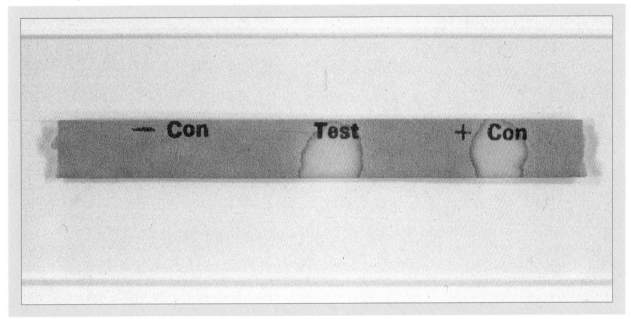

Figure 6 *Moraxella catarrhalis*: test for β-lactamase production. The importance of *Moraxella catarrhalis* (formerly *Branhamella* spp.) has only been recognized in the past few years. It is a Gram-negative coccus, and a commensal of the oropharynx. It is an opportunist pathogen particularly in patients with underlying chronic lung disease or malignancy. About 60–90% of strains produce large amounts of β-lactamase, which inactivates penicillin and ampicillin/amoxycillin. Even if *M. catarrhalis* is not actually responsible for infection in an individual, it is thought that it may interfere with penicillin therapy given for other reasons, by inactivating the antibiotic in the oropharyngeal secretions

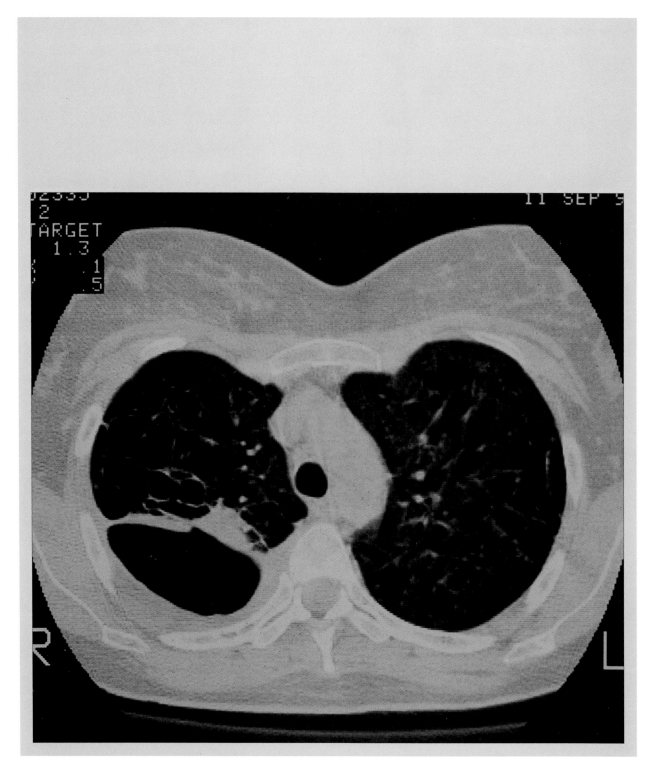

Figure 7 CT scan of the thorax of a patient with emphysema

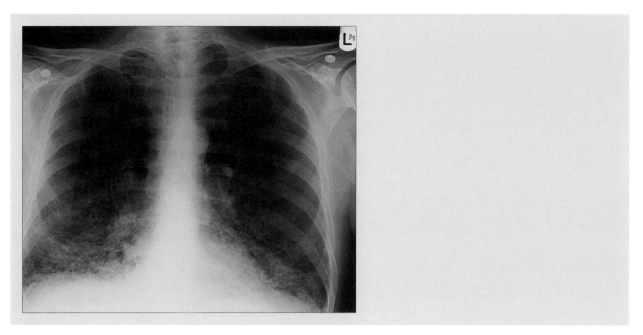

Figure 8 Chest radiograph showing bilateral basal bronchiectasis

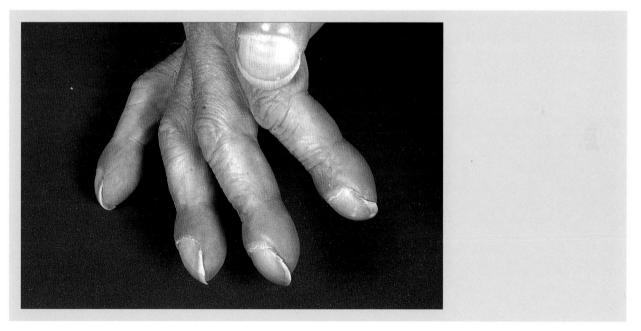

Figure 9 Finger clubbing. Clubbing is associated with bronchiectasis and pleural empyema˙

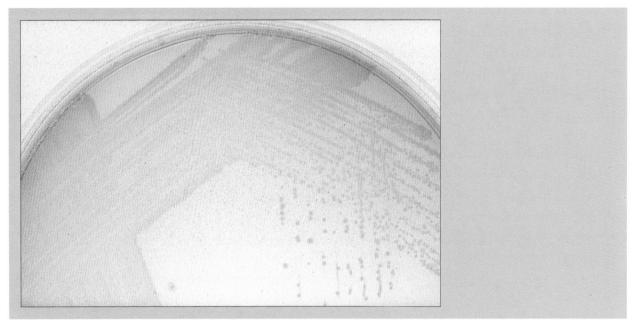

Figure 10 *Pseudomonas aeruginosa* culture on nutrient agar. *Pseudomonas* is a strict aerobe which may be cultured from the sputum of patients with bronchiectasis or cystic fibrosis. It is recognized by its distinctive green pigment (pyocyanin) and it is oxidase positive. It is frequently seen as a commensal in hospitalized patients and treatment is unnecessary unless appropriate signs and symptoms of infection are also present. Cetrimide agar can be used as a selective medium for *Pseudomonas aeruginosa*

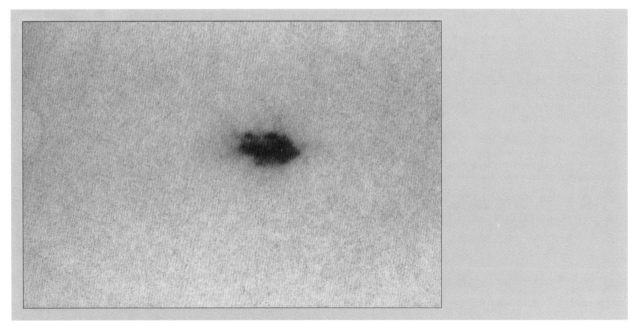

Figure 11 Oxidase test. *Pseudomonas* spp. give this purple reaction with oxidase reagent (oxidase positive), in contrast to other aerobic Gram-negative rods such as enterobacteria (e.g. *Escherichia coli* and *Klebsiella* spp.) which are oxidase negative and produce a pink reaction. The organism can therefore be presumptively identified in the laboratory as *Pseudomonas* spp. Although further tests may be needed, presumptive identification of *Pseudomonas* can be a useful guide to early antibiotic therapy, if required

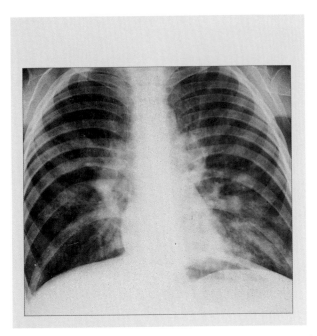

Figure 12 Cystic fibrosis in a child. Chest radiograph shows hyperinflation with bronchial wall thickening and areas of collapse

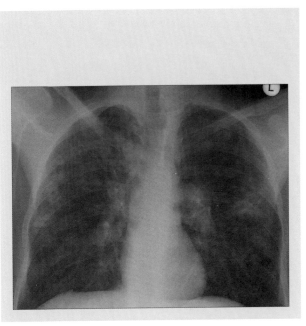

Figure 13 Cystic fibrosis in a young adult. Chest radio-graph shows prominent pulmonary vessels and a normal-sized heart. The lung fields show typical changes of bronchiectasis with ring shadows and band shadows representing chronic inflammation and thickening of the bronchiole walls. Areas of consolidation are seen in the right apex and left mid-zone

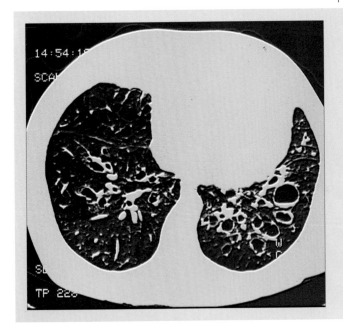

Figure 14 CT scan of the thorax of a patient with cystic fibrosis shows the dilated bronchi and fluid levels

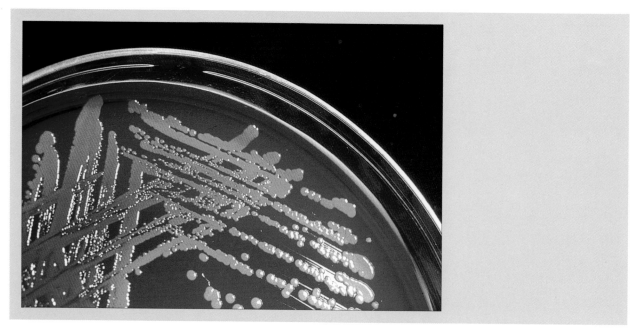

Figure 15 *Staphylococcus aureus* on blood agar. *Staphylococcus aureus* is a coagulase-positive Gram-positive coccus. It is cultured from young children with cystic fibrosis, and many pediatricians give continuous cloxacillin or flucloxacillin prophylaxis to prevent severe infection. Methicillin-resistant *Staphylococcus aureus* has become a significant problem in some centers (methicillin is used in the laboratory to test for resistance to flucloxacillin and cloxacillin)

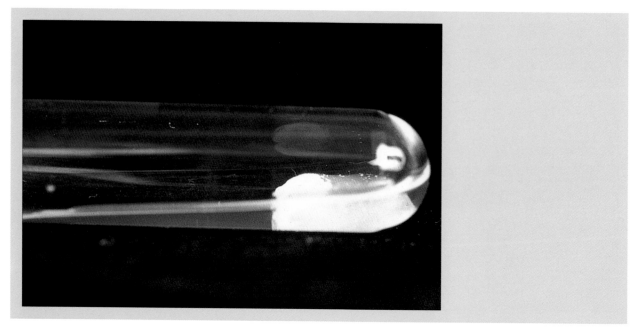

Figure 16 *Staphylococcus aureus*: tube coagulase test. If a staphylococcus is cultured from clinical specimens, it can be identified as *Staphylococcus aureus* by inoculating human plasma with a colony from the plate. Within 2–6 h, sometimes longer, *Staphylococcus aureus* causes a clot to appear (the enzyme coagulase converts fibrinogen to fibrin). Coagulase may be a virulence factor which helps to protect the organism against the host's immune responses

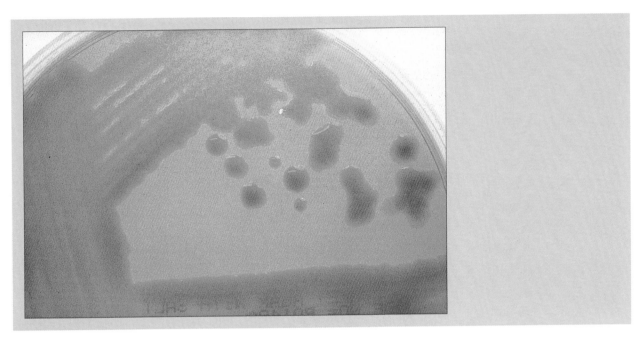

Figure 17 *Pseudomonas aeruginosa*: mucoid strain on nutrient agar. Older children and adults with cystic fibrosis are frequently colonized with strains of *Pseudomonas aeruginosa* that produce large amounts of extracellular polysaccharide, possibly enhancing resistance to host defences in the respiratory tract

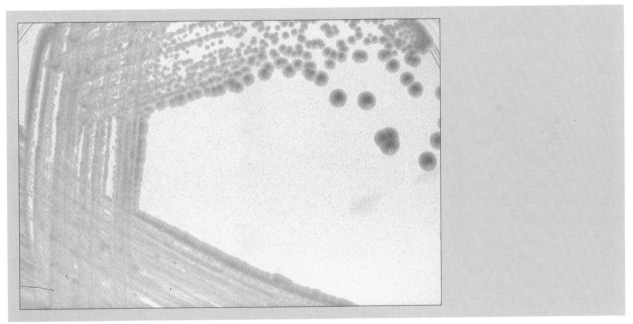

Figure 18 *Pseudomonas (Burkholderia) cepacia* on a selective medium. *Pseudomonas (Burkholderia) cepacia* has recently been recognized as an important cause of colonization or infection in patients with cystic fibrosis, and is frequently more resistant to antibiotics. It is more difficult to culture from sputum than *Ps. aeruginosa*. A selective medium (containing crystal violet and antibiotics) can improve the isolation of the organism

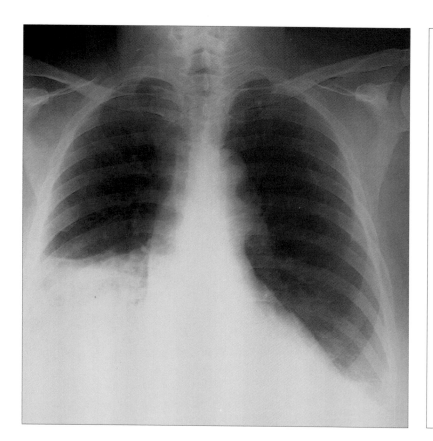

Figure 19 Pneumococcal pneumonia. Anteroposterior erect chest radiograph shows right middle and lower lobe consolidation with right-sided pleural effusion

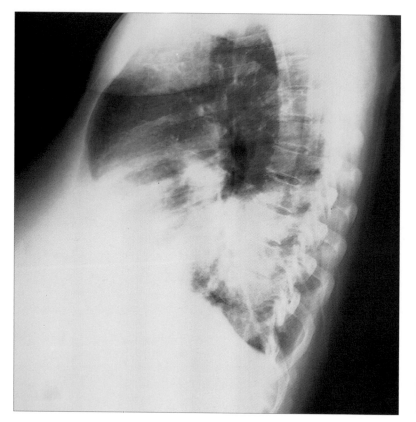

Figure 20 Pneumococcal pneumonia. Lateral chest radiograph

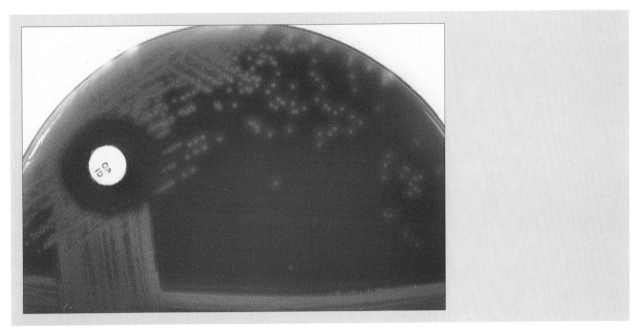

Figure 21 *Streptococcus pneumoniae*: optochin sensitivity. Streptococci cause partial degradation of blood (α-hemolysis). Cultures of respiratory tract secretions often contain viridans streptococci such as *Streptococcus salivarius* and several other species which are commensals in the oropharynx. Viridans streptococci are also α-hemolytic and so pneumococci have to be distinguished from them. Pneumococci (but not viridans streptococci or other streptococci) are sensitive to the antibiotic optochin, and a disc containing optochin is placed on the agar plate to aid identification

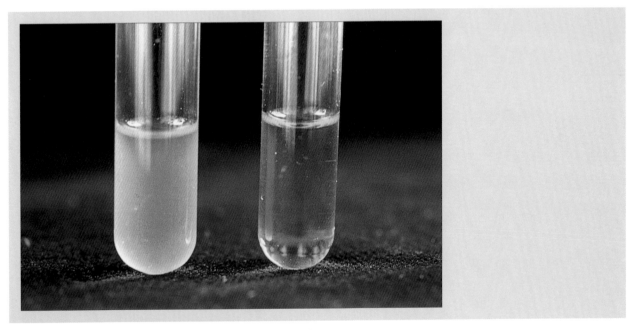

Figure 22 *Streptococcus pneumoniae*: bile solubility. *Streptococcus pneumoniae* autolyses (i.e. is 'soluble') in a solution of bile salts, unlike other streptococci. The bile salts activate an autolytic enzyme possessed by the organism. *Streptococcus pneumoniae* has been inoculated into the right-hand tube, and a viridans streptococcus into the left tube

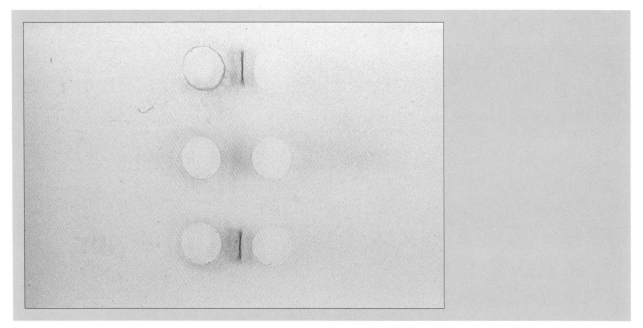

Figure 23 Countercurrent immunoelectrophoresis (CIE). CIE detects microbial antigens by using specific antisera. Serum, sputum or urine obtained from patients with septicemia or pneumonia caused by capsular pathogens such as pneumococci, haemophili and meningococci contain capsular polysaccharide, since antigen is released from the organism. To detect the capsular antigen, an agarose gel is prepared in which small wells are cut, and one is filled with the serum (or other specimen). The opposite well is filled with an antiserum to the capsular antigens of *Streptococcus pneumoniae* (antigens from other organisms such as haemophilus can also be detected if appropriate antisera are used). A 200-volt potential difference is applied across the gel, and the antigen and antibody will precipitate as a thin line between the two wells. The gel has been stained for clarity. CIE is not very sensitive and false-positives may occur. Latex agglutination or coagglutination methods are replacing CIE in many laboratories

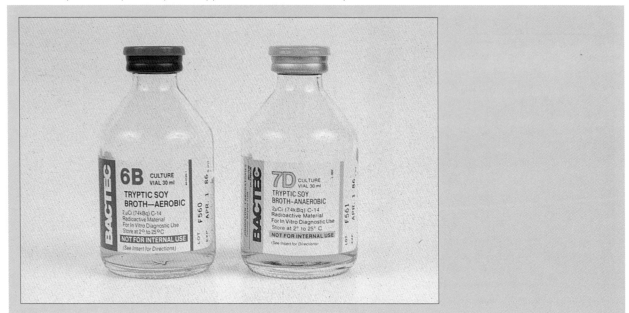

Figure 24 Blood culture set. It is essential to take blood cultures from patients with acute pneumonia. One or two blood culture sets are sufficient in most cases. There is a variety of blood culture systems; a commonly-used automated type (illustrated) detects CO_2 gas produced by growing organisms. The head space above the fluid is sampled once or twice daily and an increase in CO_2 is detected spectrophotometrically. An earlier system uses a radiolabelled carbon substrate, and radioactive CO_2 is detected. Once a bottle is positive for CO_2, the broth is Gram-stained and subcultured onto agar for further identification and measurement of sensitivities

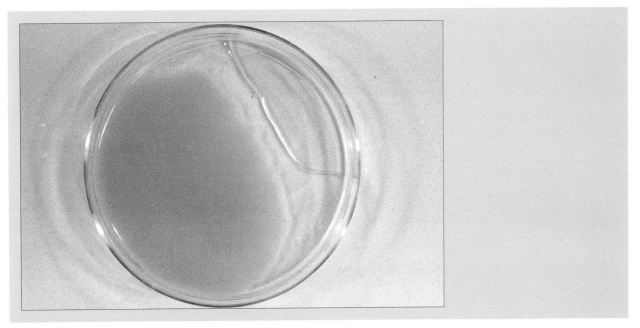

Figure 25 Purulent sputum sample, macroscopic view. Sputum samples from patients with suspected pneumonia are frequently salivary or mucoid and are of little or no value for culture. Sputum samples should be mucopurulent or purulent, and obtained by deep coughing together with physiotherapy, if necessary

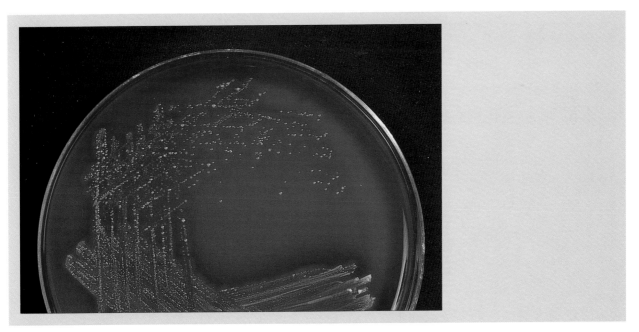

Figure 26 Culture of a sputum sample always yields a selection of the patient's normal respiratory flora. Occasionally, a pure culture of pathogens such as pneumococci or haemophili is grown but normally the culture is mixed and the pathogens must be separated to obtain pure cultures for identification and sensitivity tests. The normal flora may obscure underlying pathogens and selective agars can sometimes help to overcome this problem. The sputum of patients receiving broad-spectrum antibiotics may become colonized with coliforms, pseudomonas or yeasts but, if there is no clinical evidence of pulmonary infection, treatment is not indicated in such patients

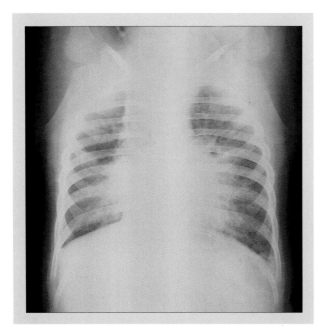

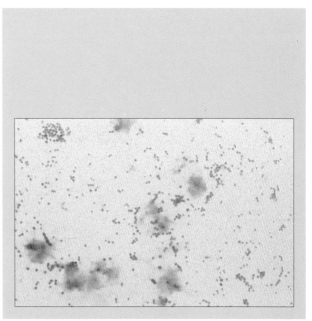

Figure 27 Staphylococcal pneumonia in a small child. Chest radiograph shows widespread bilateral infiltrates with pneumatocele formation. Volume loss, cavitation and pleural effusion or empyema are common

Figure 28 *Staphylococcus aureus* pneumonia: Gram stain of sputum × 800. *S. aureus* pneumonia may need to be considered in certain cases of community-acquired pneumonia, particularly if the patient has recently had influenza. A diagnosis of staphylococcal pneumonia may be suggested if large numbers of Gram-positive cocci in clusters are seen on a Gram stain of sputum. It should be noted that sputum normally contains a few Gram-positive cocci as part of the normal flora

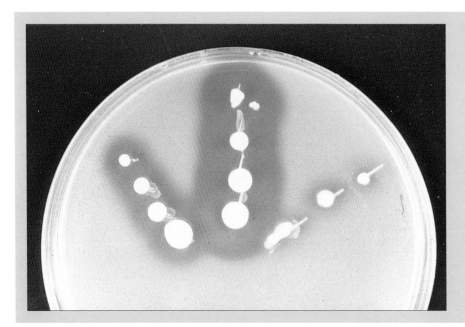

Figure 29 *Staphylococcus aureus*: DNAse test. *Staphylococcus aureus* produces DNAse as well as coagulase (Figure 16), probably as a virulence factor. The test can be used to identify the organism in the laboratory. The test organism is inoculated into agar containing calf thymus DNA, and, after incubation, the plate is flooded with hydrochloric acid which precipitates the DNA. A clear zone in the agar around the colonies indicates the organism is DNAse positive, since DNA lysed by the staphylococcal DNAse will not precipitate. A negative control, another species of staphylococcus which does not produce DNAse, is also included on the plate

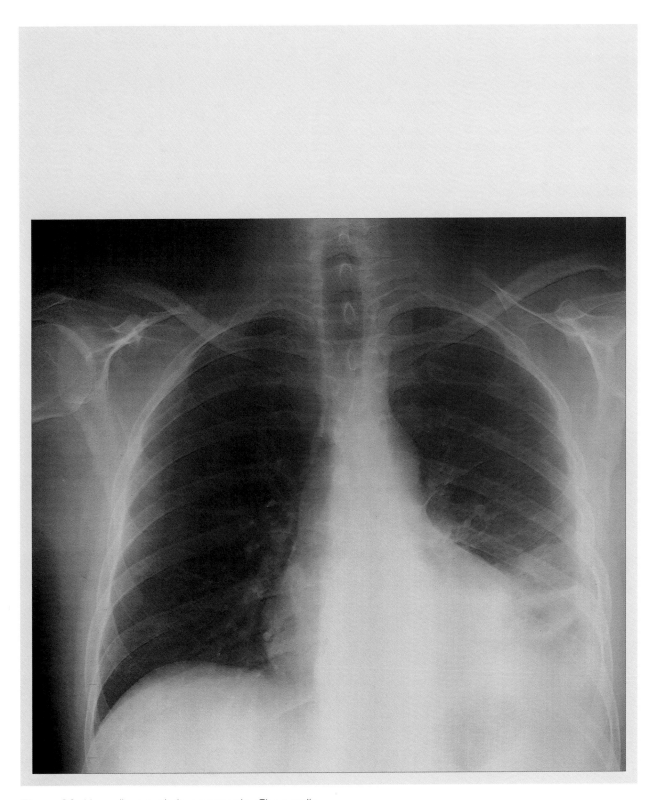

Figure 30 *Moraxella catarrhalis* pneumonia. Chest radiograph shows left lower lobe consolidation and a left pleural effusion

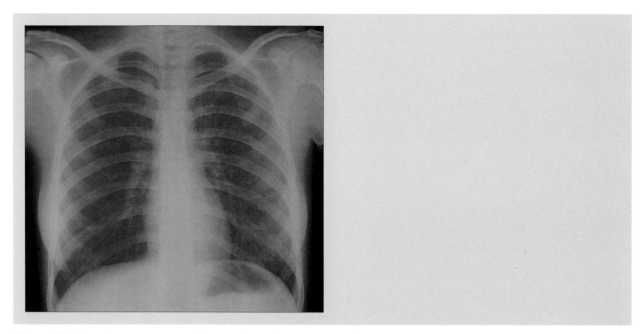

Figure 31 *Mycoplasma pneumoniae.* Chest radiograph shows a fine reticular pattern

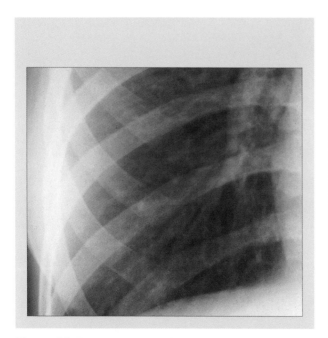

Figure 32 Enlarged section of right lower zone (normal) of chest radiograph shown in Figure 31

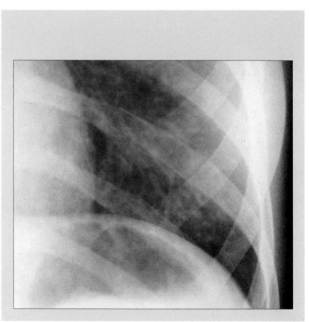

Figure 33 Enlarged section of left lower zone (abnormal) of chest radiograph shown in Figure 31

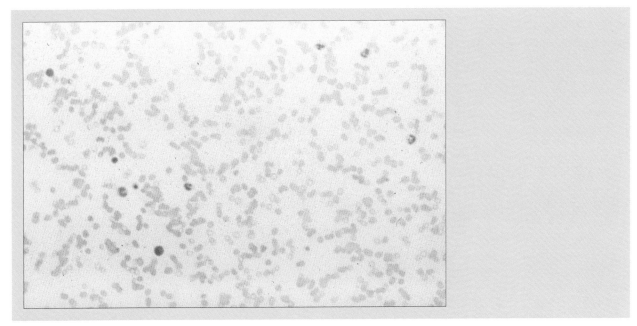

Figure 34 Cold agglutinins in a peripheral blood film (Giemsa stain × 200). Infection with *Mycoplasma pneumoniae* can often result in production of an antibody which cross-reacts at low temperatures with the 'i' antigen of human red blood cells, and causes their agglutination. 'i' antigen is similar to an antigen found on the mycoplasma cell surface. Normally, the agglutination only occurs *in vitro* at 4°C.

Agglutination is visible on a standard blood film. A tube dilution test for cold agglutinins can also be performed. The test is usually performed in conjunction with the complement fixation test for *Mycoplasma pneumoniae* to obtain a specific diagnosis, since there are other causes of cold agglutinin production

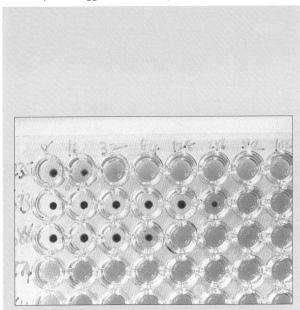

Figure 35 Complement fixation test for *Mycoplasma pneumoniae*. Because *M. pneumoniae* is very difficult to isolate from clinical specimens, diagnosis of infection is usually made by serological tests such as the complement fixation test. Some types of antibody, when bound to antigen, will fix complement. In the complement fixation test, this property is exploited. Mycoplasma antigen is added to the patient's heated serum. If antibody is present in the serum, complement (which has been added) is fixed to the antigen–antibody complex and becomes unavailable. The presence or absence of available complement therefore correlates with the absence or presence, respectively, of antibody. The indicator system (to detect any complement that has not been bound) consists of sensitized sheep red cells, i.e. sheep red cells which have been coated with an anti-sheep red cell antibody. These red cells only require complement for lysis to occur. If no lysis occurs, complement has been fixed in the first reaction, and antibody was therefore present in the patient's serum. To assess the amount of antibody present (quantified as a titer), the serum is initially diluted from 1 in 4 to 1 in 1024. The wells with a 'button' of cells at the bottom are those in which antibody has been detected, whereas complete red cell lysis occurs in wells without antibody. Serum with a high level of antibody can be diluted many times over before the reaction in the well becomes negative. If possible, two blood samples are taken from the patient a few days apart, and a fourfold or more rising titer (e.g. from a titer of 1 in 8 to 1 in 32) is taken to be a significant rise in antibody

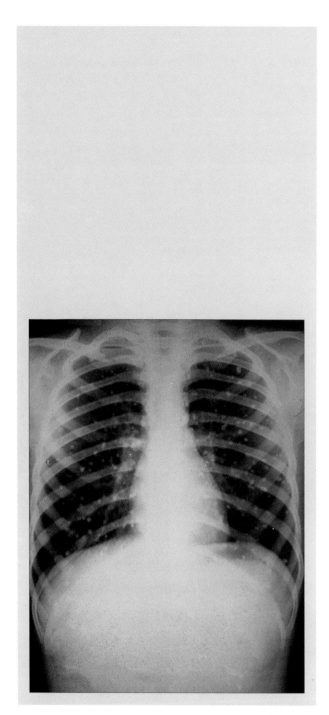

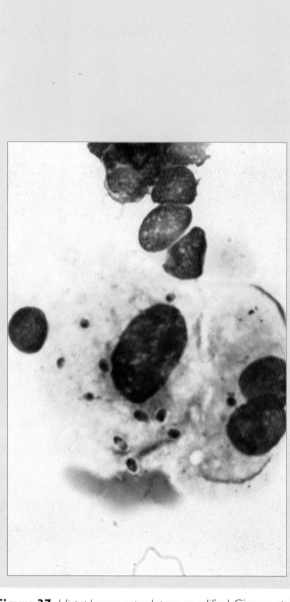

Figure 36 *Histoplasmosis.* Chest radiograph shows calcified loci in the lungs and in lymph nodes in the hilar and mediastinum

Figure 37 *Histoplasma capsulatum*: modified Giemsa stain × 1000. *Histoplasma capsulatum* is a dimorphic fungus, found in the soil. It grows as a yeast at 37°C and in a mycelial form at lower temperatures. Here the organism is seen as small oval or round yeasts within macrophages. Histoplasma can be cultured from respiratory specimens but care is needed as the organism is a laboratory hazard. For the diagnosis of histoplasmosis, serological tests are more commonly performed than culture. These include an immunodiffusion-precipitin test and a complement fixation test. Photograph courtesy of Dr W. Keith Hadley, San Francisco General Hospital

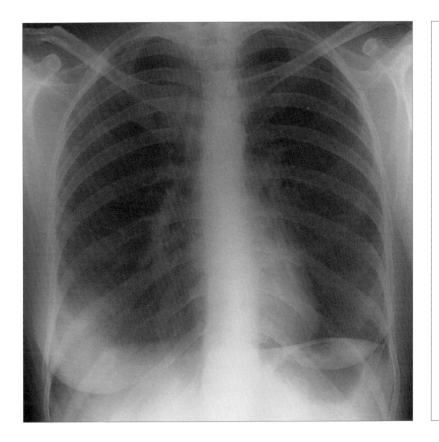

Figure 38 *Chlamydia psittaci* pneumonia. Chest radiograph shows segmental consolidation in the lateral segment of the right lower lobe

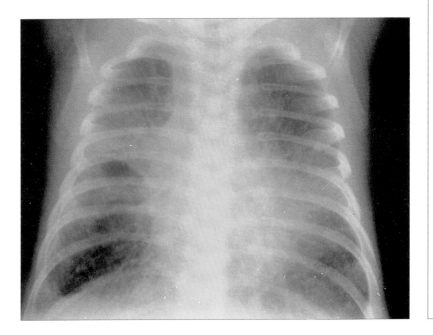

Figure 39 *Chlamydia trachomatis* pneumonia in a neonate. The radiographic appearances are variable and indistinguishable from those produced by viruses or pertussis

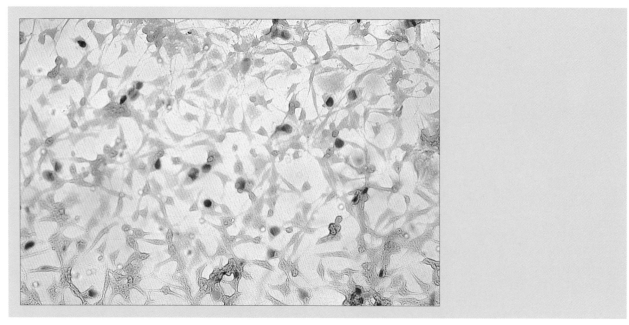

Figure 40 *Chlamydia* inclusions in cell culture (iodine stain). Chlamydiae can be grown in cell culture (irradiated McCoy cells) and stained with iodine stain or Giemsa. *Chlamydia trachomatis* (in this figure) contains glycogen and the organism takes up the iodine more readily than *C. psittaci*. Culture of *C. psittaci* is difficult and hazardous and so psittacosis is usually diagnosed by detecting a high or rising titer of antibody in the complement fixation test

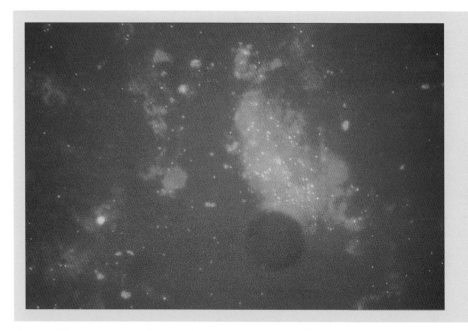

Figure 41 *Chlamydia trachomatis* immunofluorescence. *C. trachomatis* can be detected in clinical specimens by direct immunofluorescence. A smear of the clinical sample is treated with specific antibody to *C. trachomatis* which has been labelled with fluorescein. After washing, the smear is examined with an ultraviolet light microscope, and yellow-green fluorescent elementary bodies are seen. An ELISA can also be used to detect chlamydial antigen. The organism grows in irradiated McCoy cells and the intracellular bodies can be seen on light microscopy if the cells are stained with Giemsa or iodine stains. However, cell culture has been replaced by direct immunofluorescence or ELISA methods in many laboratories

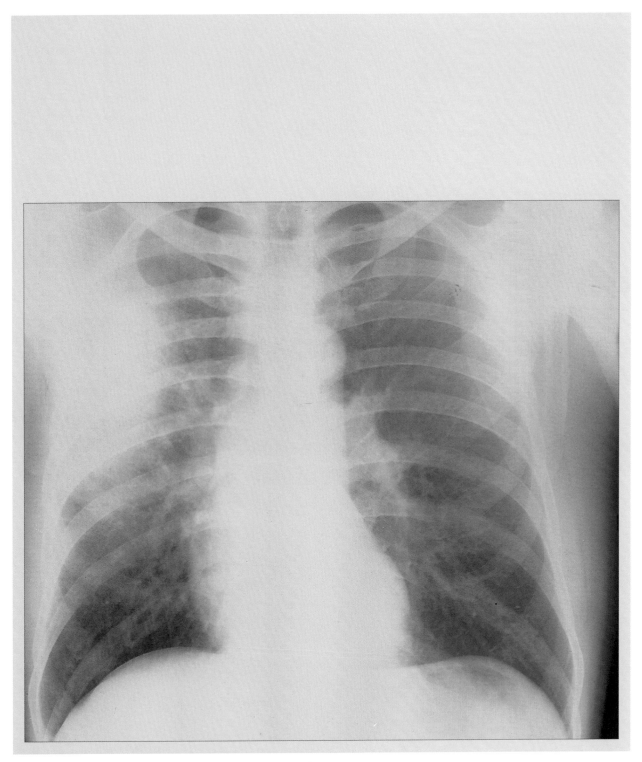

Figure 42 *Coxiella burnetii* (Q fever). Chest radiograph shows an area of consolidation which is radiologically indistinguishable from other atypical pneumonias

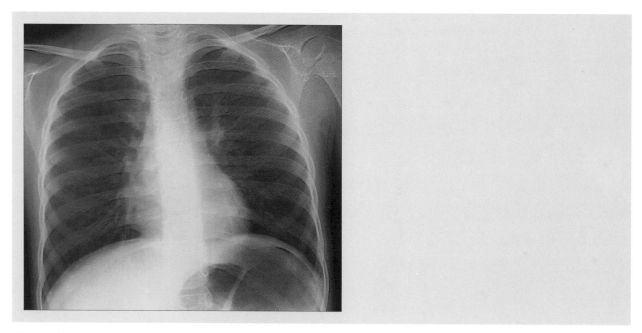

Figure 43 Respiratory syncytial virus. Chest radiograph shows diffuse air trapping, indicated by hyperinflation and low, flat diaphragms. Peribronchial thickening produces ring shadows or parallel linear shadows

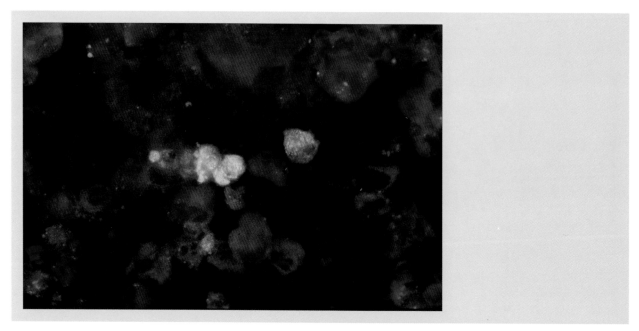

Figure 44 Immunofluorescence of respiratory syncytial virus (RSV) in a nasopharyngeal aspirate. Direct immunofluorescence uses specific antibody (in this case antibody to RSV), to which a fluorescein molecule has been linked. Nasopharyngeal secretions from a child with suspected RSV bronchiolitis are inoculated onto a slide and the labelled antibody is added; the slide is then washed. When the cells are examined with an ultraviolet microscope, fluorescence is seen in those cells infected with RSV. This type of immunofluorescence can be used for other viruses, such as influenza and parainfluenza viruses, provided the appropriate labelled antibody is used

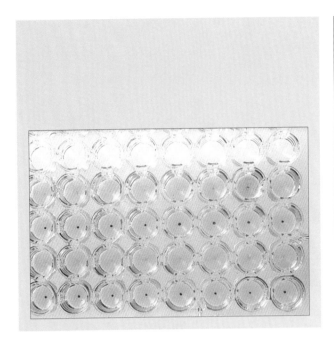

Figure 45 Hemagglutination inhibition test for anti-bodies to influenza virus. The principle of this test rests on the ability of some viruses (e.g. influenza and rubella) to hemagglutinate red cells; antibody prevents this agglutination. Standard amounts of virus are added to the patient's serum, which has been prepared in a range of dilutions. Chick red cells are then added to each well. If antibody is present in the serum, it binds to the virus and prevents the cells hemagglutinating; they settle as a button at the bottom of the well. If no antibody is present, a thin layer of red cells forms. In the figure, the first and third sera contain a high titer of antibody whereas the other two contain none. It should be noted that some sera inhibit hemagglutination of red cells non-specifically; all sera are therefore pretreated to remove these non-specific factors. A control well is also included which has no viral antigen to ensure that the red cells do not hemagglutinate non-specifically. The test takes 6–7 h and is used principally for rubella, but occasionally for influenza, mumps and adenoviruses

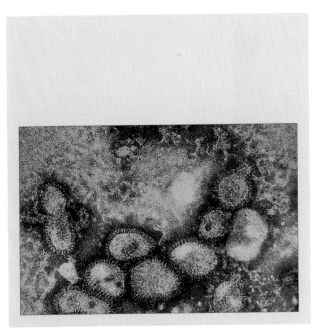

Figure 46 Electron micrograph of influenza virus. The virus is 80–120 nm in diameter. Influenza virus types A, B and C have surface projections of hemagglutinin and neuraminidase which enable the virus to bind to host cells. Influenza is normally diagnosed in the laboratory by immunofluorescence, viral culture or by detecting a rising titer of antibody in the complement fixation or hemagglutination-inhibition tests

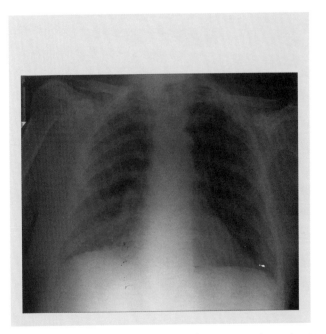

Figure 47 *Influenza pneumonia.* Anteroposterior chest radiograph shows right lower zone consolidation

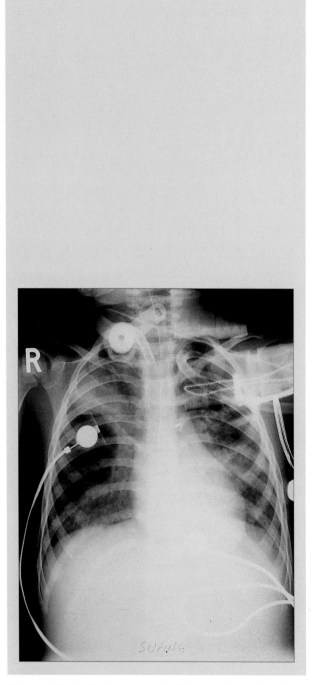

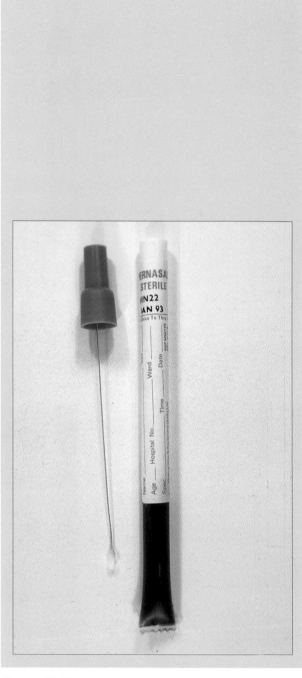

Figure 48 *Bordetella pertussis*. Chest radiograph shows bronchial wall thickening, consolidation with areas of atelectasis and an endotracheal tube

Figure 49 Pernasal swab for the diagnosis of whooping cough. *Bordetella pertussis* can be cultured from the nasopharynx, particularly in the first 2–3 weeks of the illness and less frequently thereafter. A thin-wire calcium alginate swab is passed along the floor of the nasal cavity to the pharynx. The swab is then inoculated onto Bordet–Gengou medium containing starch and charcoal or blood, and the plate incubated in high humidity for 5–7 days. The organism is identified by its colonial morphology and agglutination on a glass slide with specific antiserum to *B. pertussis*

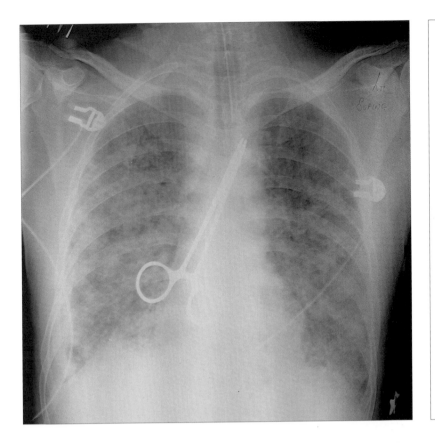

Figure 50 Varicella zoster viral pneumonia. Chest radiograph of a patient with a fatal outcome

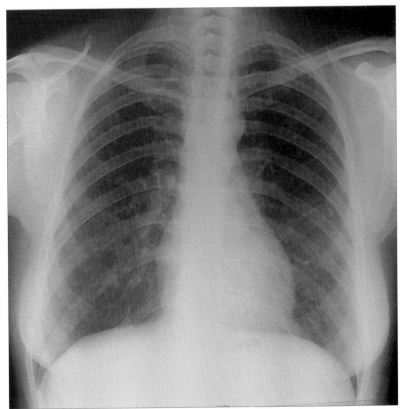

Figure 51 Varicella zoster viral pneumonia. Chest radiograph of a mild infection shows multiple small nodules in both lungs

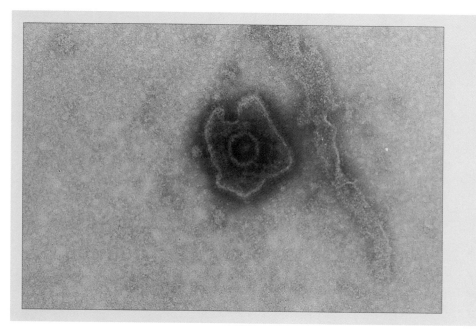

Figure 52 Electron micrograph of varicella zoster virus. If a patient with suspected varicella pneumonia has skin lesions, urgent electron microscopy of vesicle fluid from the skin should be performed. The vesicle fluid is smeared on a glass slide, and the area marked with a pen on the other side of the slide. A swab can also be taken from the vesicle, placed in viral transport medium and cultured for varicella zoster virus and herpes simplex virus. It is not possible to distinguish between herpes simplex virus and varicella zoster virus on electron microscopy. To distinguish between them, a swab should be taken from the vesicle, placed in viral transport medium and cultured for herpesviruses. The virus (nucleocapsid plus envelope) is 150–250 nm across. The nucleocapsid is 100 nm across

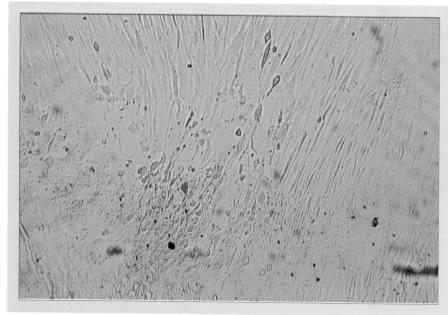

Figure 53 Cell culture of varicella zoster virus. Direct electron microscopy examination of respiratory secretions for herpesviruses is not useful, but bronchial lavage fluid and skin lesions can be cultured in suspected varicella zoster virus or herpes simplex pneumonia. Both these viruses grow rapidly in fibroblast cell culture, and a cytopathic effect is seen within 2–3 days. Immunofluorescence (labelled antibody to varicella zoster virus and herpes simplex virus) can be performed on fluid taken from the cell culture

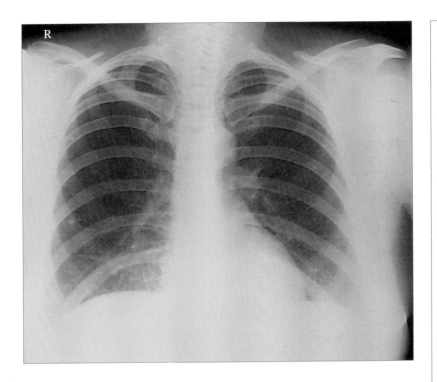

Figure 54 Calcified varicella zoster pneumonia. Chest radiograph shows calcification of the mid to lower zone, with nodules usually less than 3 mm in diameter

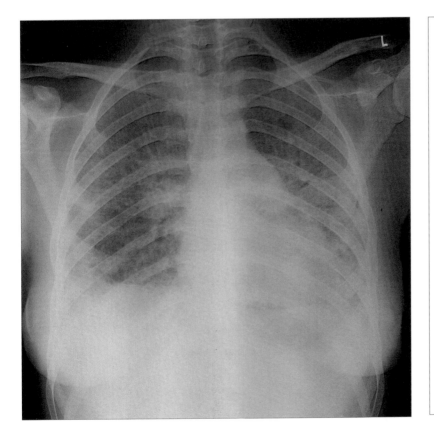

Figure 55 Measles (giant cell) pneumonia. Chest radiograph shows widespread primary viral pneumonia with extensive bilateral confluent shadowing and a right pleural effusion. The left pulmonary artery is prominent due to an atrial septal defect repair at 18 years of age

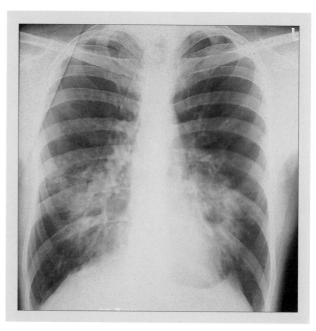

Figure 57 Chest radiograph shows fleeting bilateral shadows of allergic bronchopulmonary aspergillosis

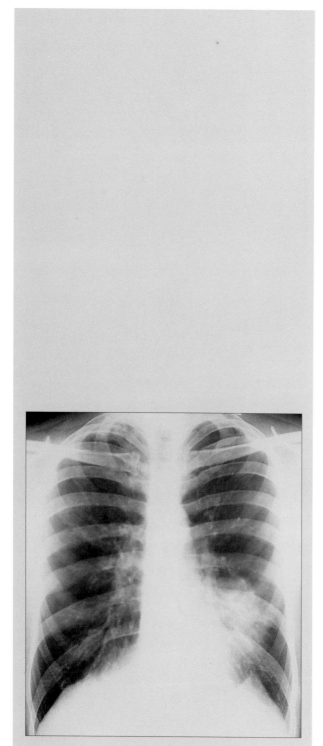

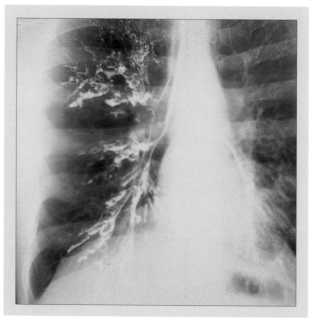

Figure 56 Allergic bronchopulmonary aspergillosis. Chest radiograph shows the acute phase with left-sided shadowing

Figure 58 Bronchogram in a patient with allergic bronchopulmonary aspergillosis showing proximal bronchiectasis

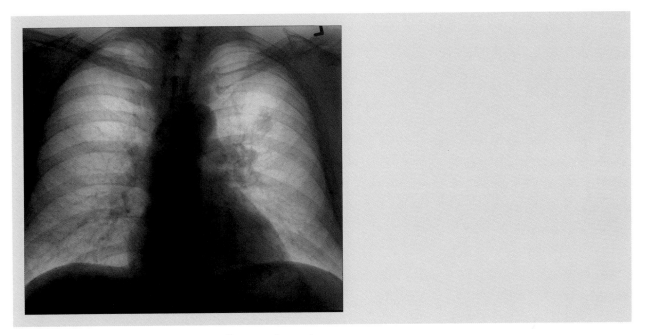

Figure 59 Acute coccidioidomycosis. Chest radiograph shows left mid-zone infiltrate associated with left hilar lymphadenopathy

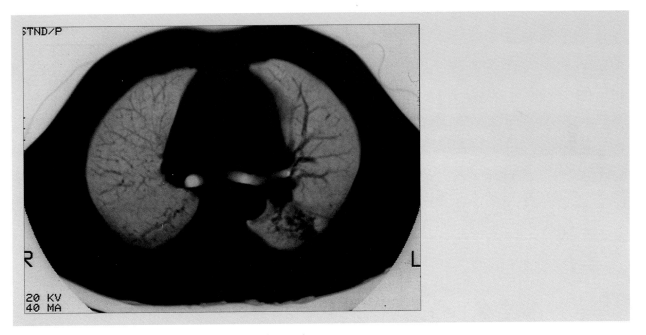

Figure 60 Acute coccidioidomycosis. CT scan shows the lesion to be abutting on the pleura and to contain an area of necrosis. Large left hilar nodes are visible. Film courtesy of Dr Jeffrey Klein, San Francisco General Hospital and Professor Phillip C. Hopewell, University of California, San Francisco

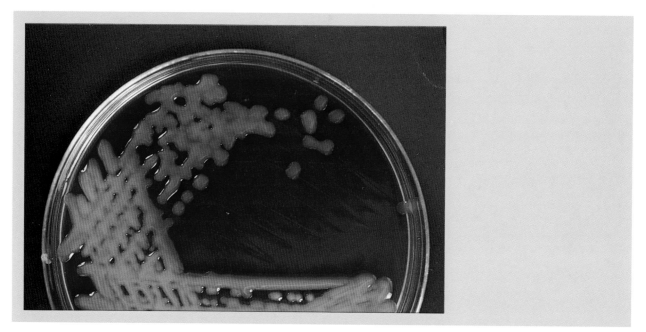

Figure 61 *Klebsiella pneumoniae* on MacConkey agar. Klebsiella, together with other enterobacteria (coliforms), can cause severe and life-threatening opportunistic infection. It is easily grown in the laboratory, and has a mucoid appearance. Its presence in sputum does not necessarily indicate infection, particularly if there are no clinical or radiological signs. Outbreaks of infection caused by multiply-resistant klebsiellae are sometimes seen on intensive care units

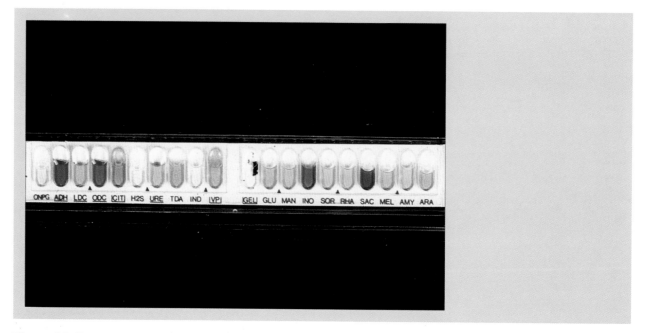

Figure 62 Biochemical identification of enterobacteria. Laboratories commonly use commercially available systems such as the API-20E (BioMerieux) to identify enterobacteria such as *Klebsiella* spp. A colony of the organism is taken from the culture plate and a suspension of it is inoculated into a tray containing a series of biochemical tests. After overnight incubation, the reactions are read and the organism is identified from a database of identity profiles

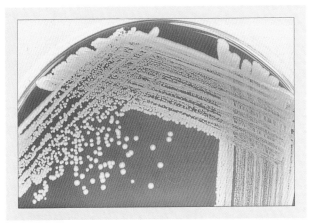

Figure 64 *Staphylococcus epidermidis* on blood agar. *Staphylococcus epidermidis* is one of the coagulase-negative staphylococci (see Figure 16). It is commonly found colonizing the respiratory tract of ventilated infants and rarely causes infection. However, repeated isolation from blood cultures of a strain of *Staphylococcus epidermidis* with an antibiogram similar to the isolate in the respiratory tract, together with relevant clinical and radiological signs, suggests that lung infection due to this organism is present. Infection is more likely in infants of very low birth weight, and often it is resistant to most anti-staphylococcal antibiotics except vancomycin

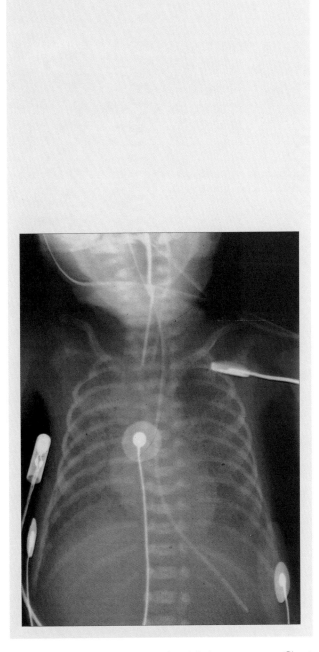

Figure 63 *Staphylococcus epidermidis* in a neonate. Chest radiograph shows a ground-glass appearance consistent with the diagnosis and right upper zone consolidation

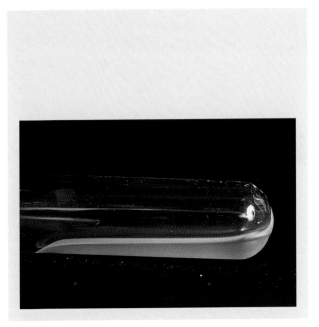

Figure 65 *Staphylococcus epidermidis*: coagulase test. In contrast to *Staphylococcus aureus*, no fibrin clot is seen when *Staphylococcus epidermidis* is incubated with plasma at 37°C for 2 or more hours

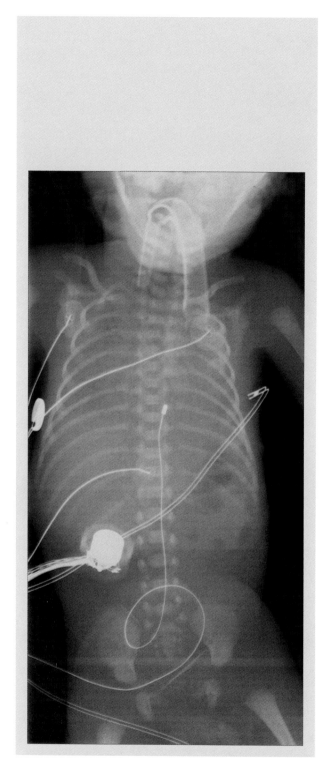

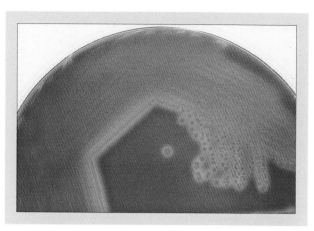

Figure 67 Group B streptococcus on blood agar. Group B streptococcus (*Streptococcus agalactiae*) is an important pathogen of neonates and infants up to the age of about 3 months. The organism is normally acquired from the mother's vaginal flora, although late-onset infection (after 10 days of age) can be acquired from other close contacts. In early-onset pneumonia and septicemia, the organism is readily cultured from superficial swabs, blood cultures and gastric aspirate. Severe group B streptococcal disease is occasionally seen in adult intensive care patients and intravenous drug users

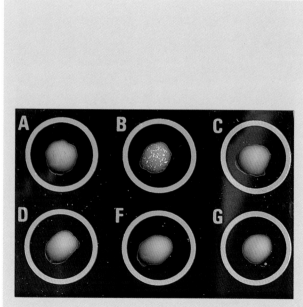

Figure 66 Group B streptococcus in a neonate. Chest radiograph shows confluent opacification with air bronchograms and the loss of all mediastinal and diaphragmatic borders

Figure 68 Group B streptococcus identification. To identify the group B streptococcus, and other streptococci, specific antisera bound to latex particles are mixed with an extract of the organism. A similar technique can be used to detect directly streptococcal antigens in body fluids

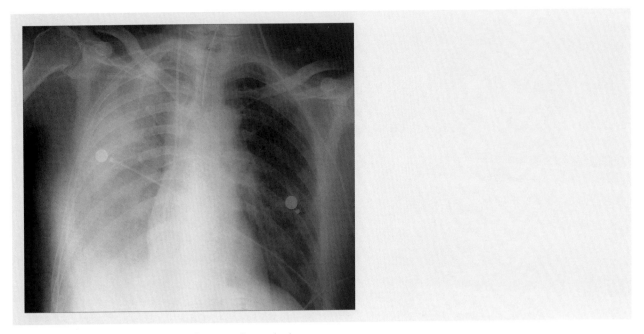

Figure 69 Legionella pneumonia. Chest radiograph shows consolidation in the right lung in a ventilated patient

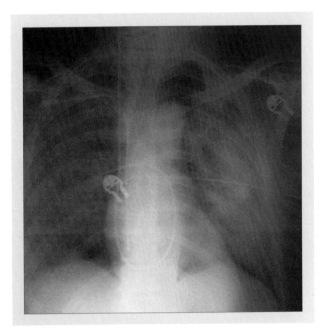

Figure 70 Chest radiograph shows spread to involve both lung fields in the same patient as in Figure 71. A Swan–Ganz catheter is *in situ*

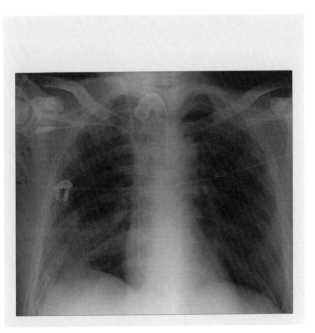

Figure 71 Chest radiograph shows marked improvement in consolidation in the same patient as in Figures 69 and 70

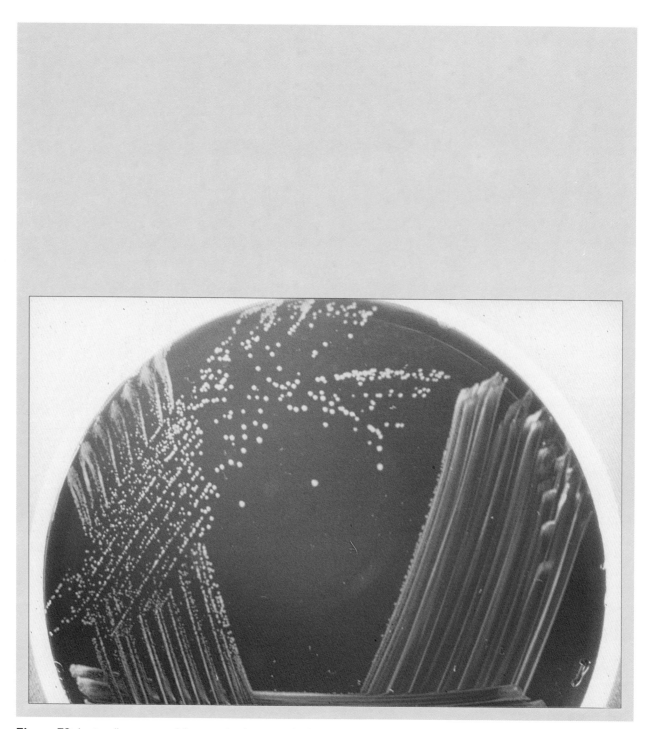

Figure 72 *Legionella pneumophila* on selective agar. Antibodies to *Legionella pneumophila* may not appear in the blood for weeks after the onset of infection (Legionnaires' disease, Pontiac fever or milder infections). An earlier diagnosis can be obtained if bronchial lavage fluid is cultured on a selective iron-rich medium. The organism will grow in 2–5 days. *L. pneumophila* serotype 1 is the most common isolate from patients with legionellosis, but other serotypes and species (e.g. *L. longbeacheae, L. bozemanii*) are sometimes grown

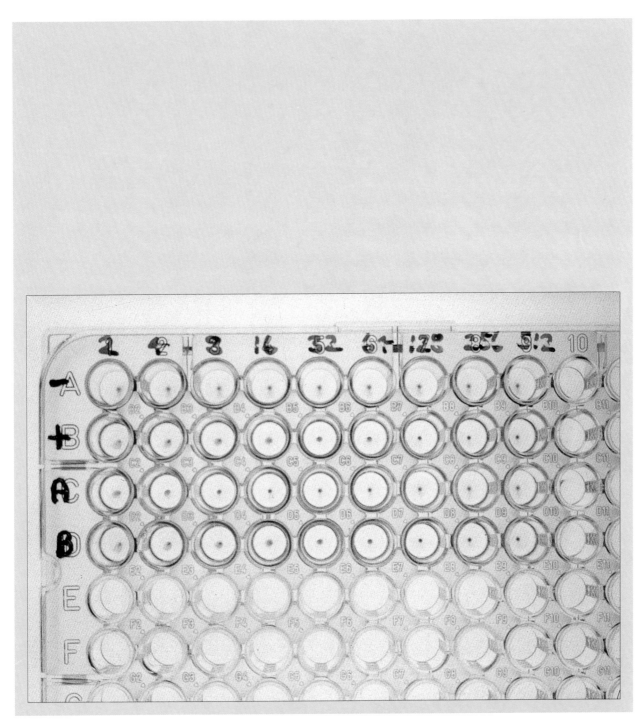

Figure 73 *Legionella pneumophila* serogroup 1: rapid micro-agglutination titer (RMAT). A titer of 1 in 8 or more in the appropriate clinical setting suggests a diagnosis of legionellosis. The diagnosis can be confirmed by repeating the test to detect a rising titer, and by performing the confirmatory immunofluorescent antibody test. A small proportion of the population has low levels of antibody to legionellae, which may be due to cross-reactivity with other organisms, or previous subclinical infection with legionellae. In the RMAT test, legionellae (stained pink) have been incubated with the patient's serum and then centrifuged and tilted at an angle. If antibody is present, a tight 'button' is formed; if not, the organisms are not bound by antibody and they spread in a line or 'teardrop' shape along the bottom of the well. In the immunofluorescent antibody test, legionellae fixed to a glass slide are exposed to the patient's serum and antibody, if present, binds to the organisms. A fluorescein-labelled anti-human antibody is then added, and, if antibody is present in the patient's serum, the organisms will be seen to fluoresce when examined with an ultraviolet light microscope

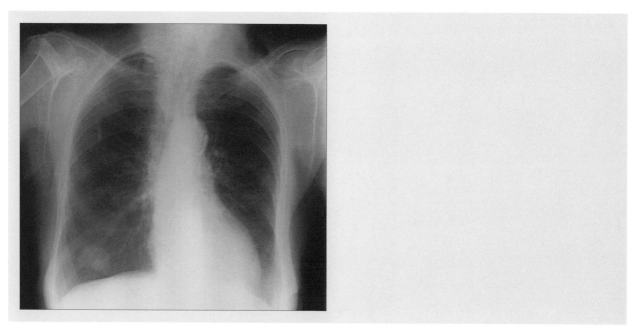

Figure 74 Nocardia. Chest radiograph shows a solitary lesion in right lower zone with patchy consolidation in the right upper zone

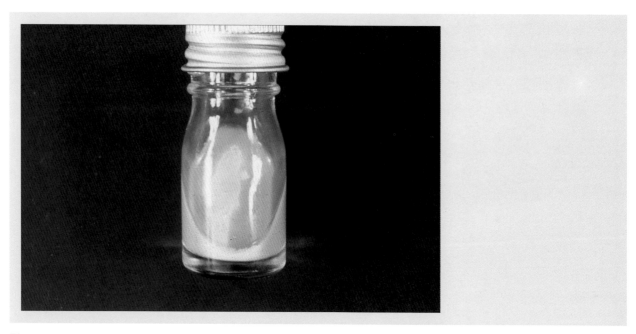

Figure 75 *Nocardia asteroides* cultured on Lowenstein–Jensen medium. Nocardia may be cultured from broncho-alveolar lavage fluid, sputum and pus on a variety of media including blood agar, Sabouraud's agar and Lowenstein–Jensen medium. The colonies become visible within 3–21 days and are often pigmented

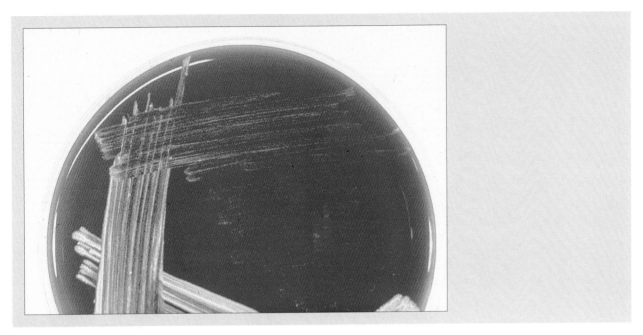

Figure 76 *Nocardia asteroides* cultured on blood agar. After 48 h culture, the colonies are tiny and may be mistaken for coryneforms (diphtheroids)

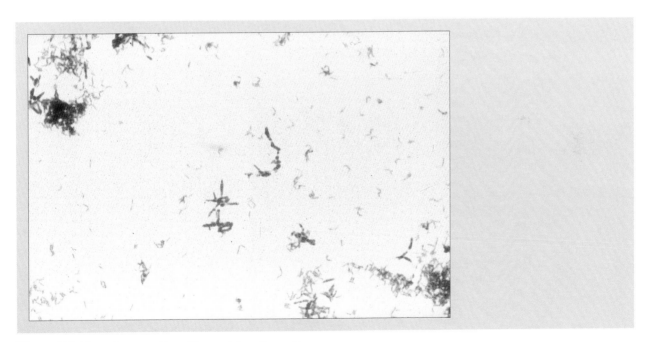

Figure 77 *Nocardia asteroides*: Gram stain of a culture. Nocardias are branching Gram-positive rods which are slightly acid-fast when a modified Ziehl–Neelsen stain is used. In clinical samples, the bacteria are more filamentous

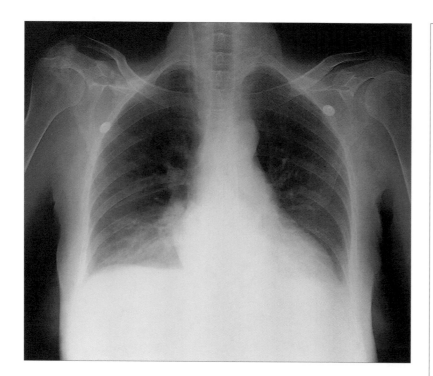

Figure 78 Cytomegalovirus pneumonia. Chest radiograph taken postoperatively in a patient given an orthotopic liver transplant for primary biliary cirrhosis. The radiograph shows consolidation of the right middle lobe

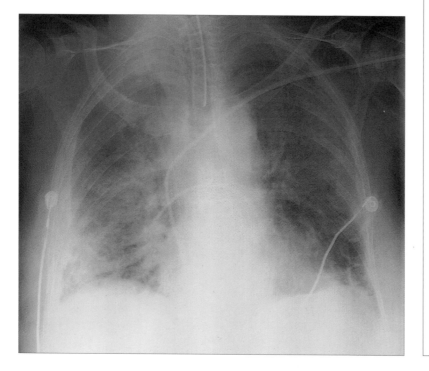

Figure 79 Two weeks later the chest radiograph of the same patient as in Figure 78 shows extensive bilateral infiltrates

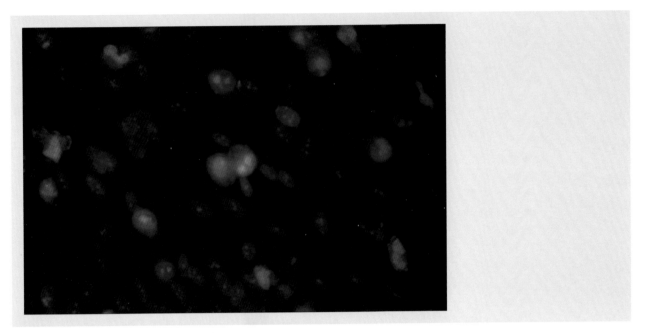

Figure 80 Cytomegalovirus: detection of early antigenic fluorescent foci (DEAFF test). Clinical samples are first inoculated into a cell culture. After 48 h, the cell culture is exposed to fluorescein-labelled antibodies, which bind to early antigens of cytomegalovirus and fluoresce when viewed under an ultraviolet light microscope

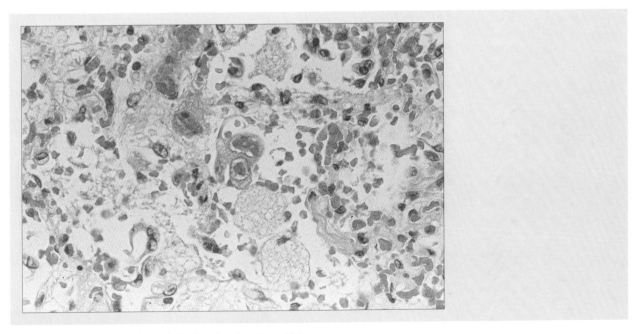

Figure 81 Cytomegalovirus: inclusion bodies in a histological section of lung: hematoxylin & eosin × 800. The section shows the typical 'owl's eye' inclusion body of cytomegalovirus

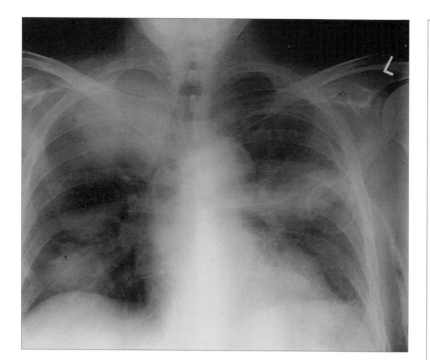

Figure 82 Disseminated invasive pulmonary aspergillosis. Chest radiograph shows typical non-specific patchy consolidation with multiple large nodules

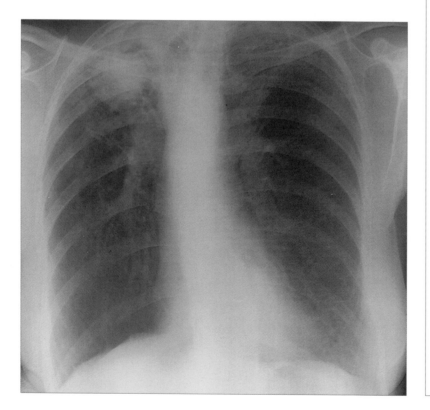

Figure 83 Aspergilloma in an old tuberculous cavity. The chest radiograph shows bilateral apical fibrosis with a cavitating mass on the right

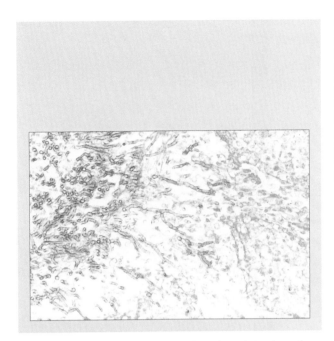

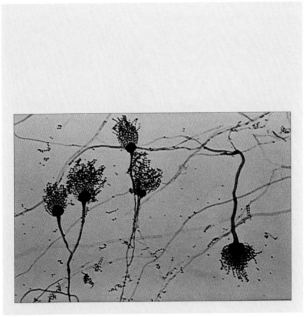

Figure 84 *Aspergillus* spp.: invasive fungal hyphae in a histological section of lung. Methenamine silver stain × 800. Invasive hyphae such as in this example are usually seen in specimens taken at postmortem

Figure 85 *Aspergillus* spp.: microscopy of a colony from a culture plate. Lactophenol cotton blue stain × 200. The characteristic fruiting bodies (macroconidia) of aspergillus are only seen in preparations from the culture plate. In clinical specimens, 'fungal elements' (mycelial forms) are seen

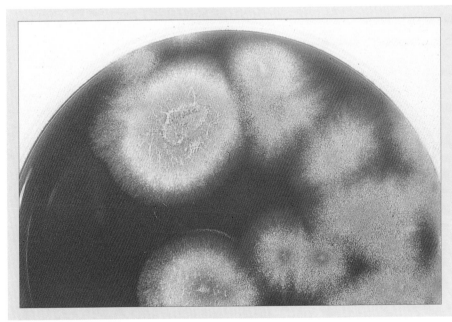

Figure 86 *Aspergillus fumigatus* growing on Sabouraud's agar. Fungal colonies usually appear on cultures of broncho-alveolar lavage fluid and other specimens within 3–5 days, but some strains take longer. Culture of *Aspergillus fumigatus* from sputum does not necessarily indicate infection but repeated isolation from sputum, or culture from the sputum of severely immunosuppressed patients, indicates probable infection

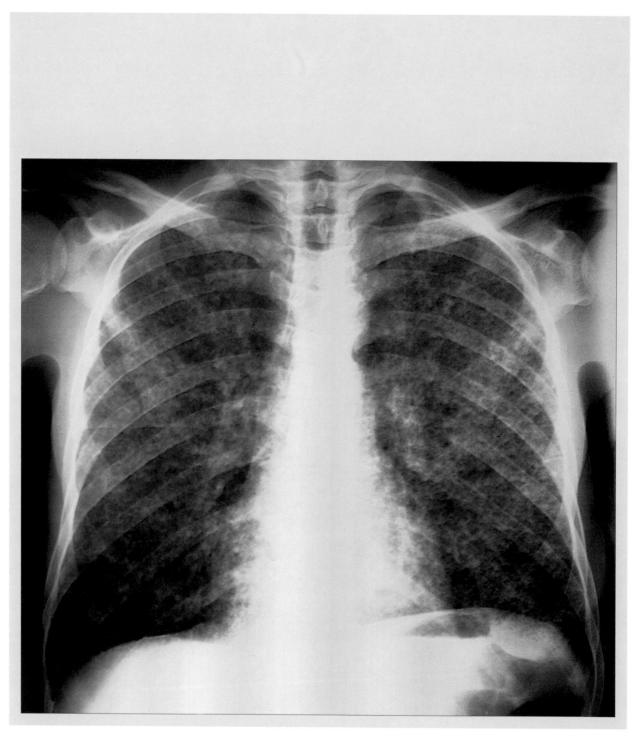

Figure 87 Strongyloides hyperinfection syndrome. Chest radiograph shows extensive reticulonodular shadowing

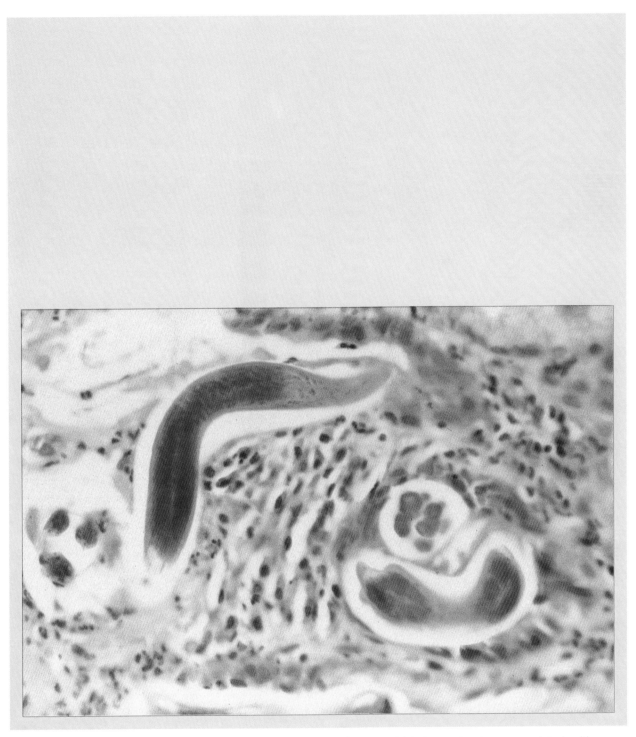

Figure 88 *Strongyloides stercoralis* in a histological section of lymph node. Hematoxylin & eosin × 800. Strongyloides is a nematode (roundworm), 0.7–2.0 mm in length, which resides in the small bowel and releases larvae into the lumen. These larvae then penetrate the skin of a new host, enter the lungs and are coughed up and swallowed. Strongyloides can survive for decades in the gut as it is also one of the few human worms that can complete its life cycle within the same host. In strongyloides hyperinfection syndrome, which is nearly always associated with some degree of immunosuppression, large numbers of larvae invade the host and are seen in the feces during life, and in biopsies or from samples taken postmortem. Stools should therefore be sent for examination for these parasites in all immunocompromised patients with unexplained fevers, if the patient has ever lived in a country where strongyloides is endemic (mainly the tropics)

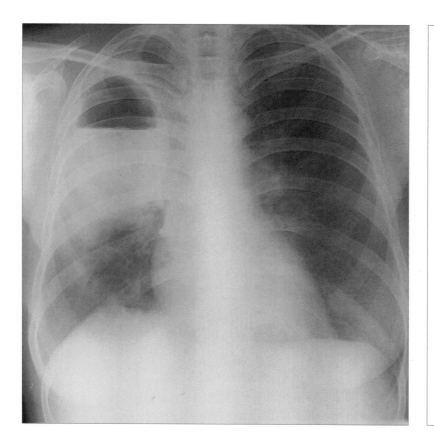

Figure 89 Staphylococcal abscess. Chest radiograph shows large abscess in the right upper lobe

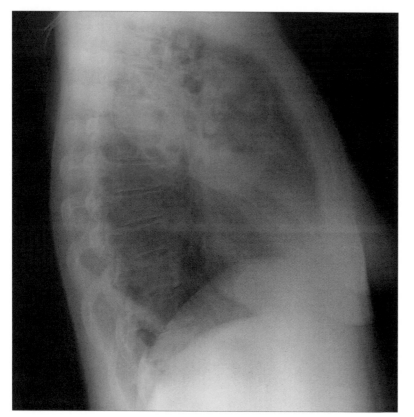

Figure 90 Staphylococcal abscess on right lateral radiograph

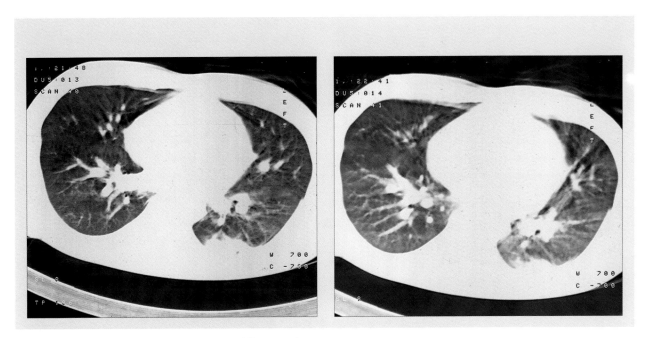

Figure 91 *Streptococcus milleri* abscesses. CT scans show cavitation of basal consolidation

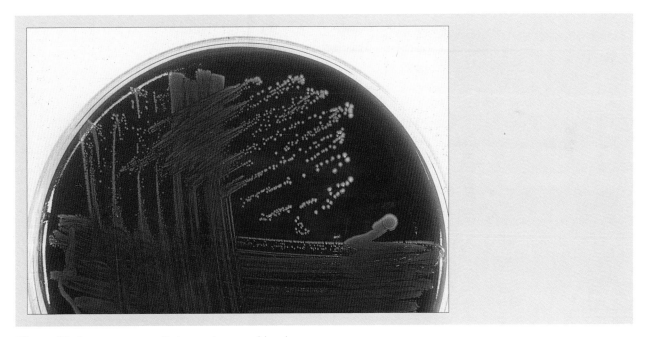

Figure 92 *Streptococcus milleri* growing on blood agar. *Streptococcus milleri* (*Streptococcus intermedius*) is easily cultured on blood agar. Many strains possess Group F Lancefield antigen, and the culture has a distinctive caramel smell

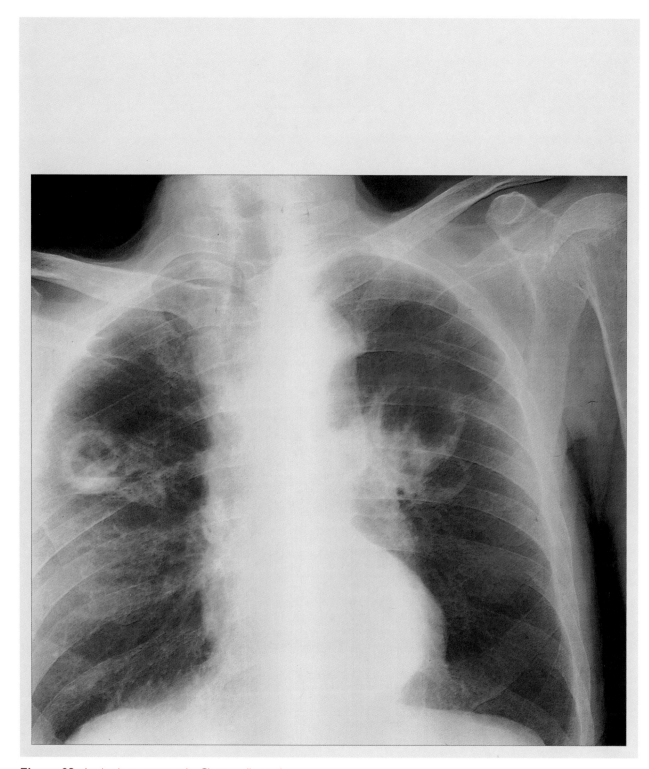

Figure 93 Aspiration pneumonia. Chest radiograph

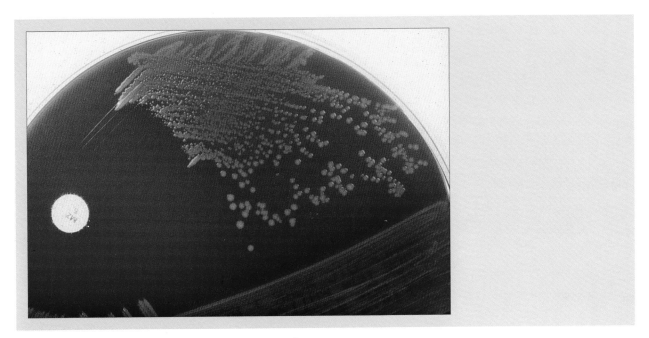

Figure 94 *Bacteroides fragilis* growing on blood agar incubated anaerobically. *Bacteroides fragilis* is the most common anaerobe isolated from human infections and is more pathogenic than other anaerobes

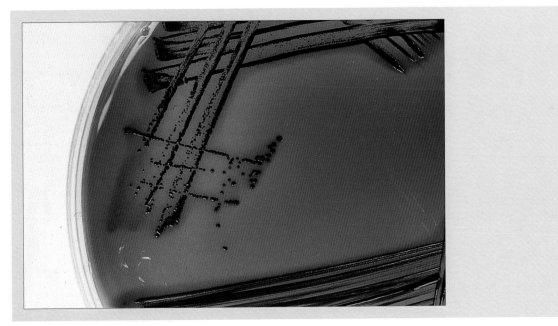

Figure 95 *Prevotella melaninogenicus* growing on blood agar incubated anaerobically. *Prevotella (Bacteroides) melaninogenicus* is a common isolate from anaerobic pus obtained from a lung abscess or pleural empyema. In pulmonary infections, the organism most probably comes from the oral flora which may have been inhaled. The colonies have a distinctive black pigmentation (the species name is a misnomer as this color is not due to melanin)

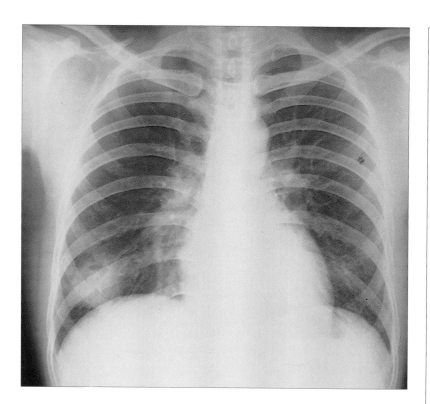

Figure 96 Hydatid cyst. Chest radiograph shows a rounded area of consolidation in the right lower zone and some air is visible in the lesion

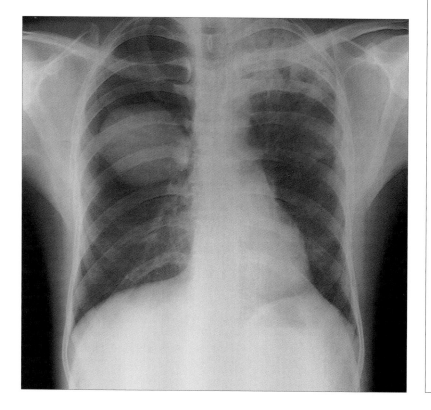

Figure 97 Hydatid cyst. In addition, chest radiograph shows findings consistent with left apical tuberculosis. The large lobulated cyst on the right is an incidental finding

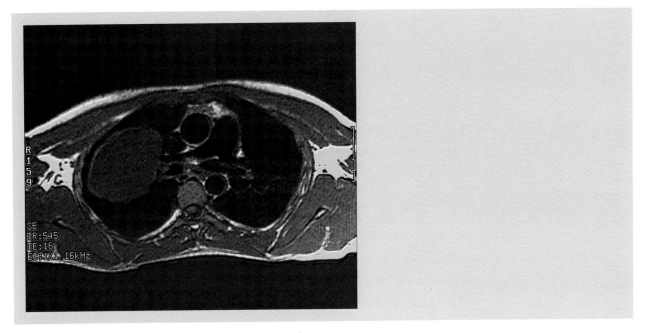

Figure 98 Magnetic resonance image of the same patient as in Figure 97 shows a well-defined fluid-filled cyst

Figure 99 Hooklet of *Echinococcus granulosus* in an aspirate of a hydatid cyst. Unstained wet mount preparation × 150. It is inadvisable to attempt needle aspiration of hydatid cysts because of the risk of dissemination of scolices. Also, the patient may have an anaphylactic reaction to hydatid proteins. Excised liver or lung cysts may be aspirated and examined for scolices or hooklets, and occasionally an abscess-like lesion may unexpectedly be found to be a hydatid cyst. The life cycle of *Echinococcus granulosus* includes canines and sheep, and man is an accidental host. Infection occurs after ingestion of hydatid ova from the feces of an infected canine. The larvae hatch from the ova and migrate to the lung, liver or other tissues and form cysts in sheep; these cysts are consumed by the canine, and the tapeworm develops in the gut, releasing ova to complete the cycle. Humans may ingest ova, and cysts are formed, but the life cycle is not completed. Serological tests, such as the hydatid complement fixation test or immunoelectrophoretic studies, should be performed if lung or liver lesions are detected in patients from areas endemic for hydatid disease, before surgery or biopsy is attempted

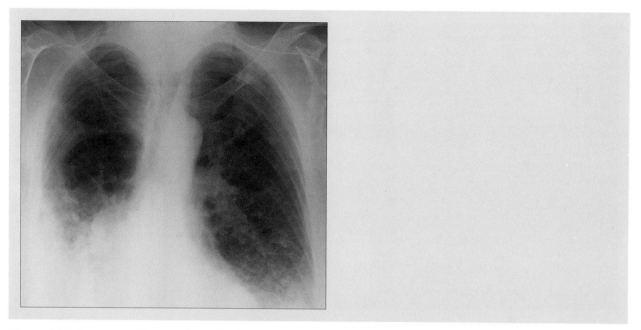

Figure 100 Empyema. Chest radiograph shows a large right-sided pleural effusion with hyperinflation and bullae in the right upper zone

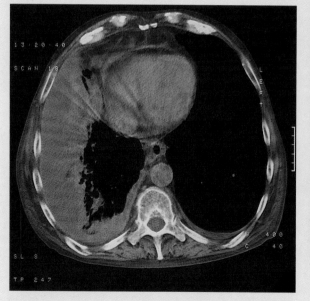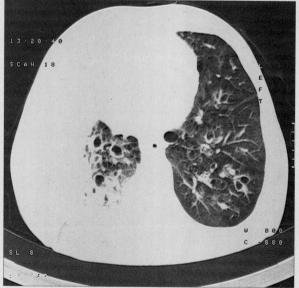

Figure 101 CT scans of the thorax of the same patient as in Figure 100 demonstrate the volume of the empyema and pre-existing bronchial wall damage

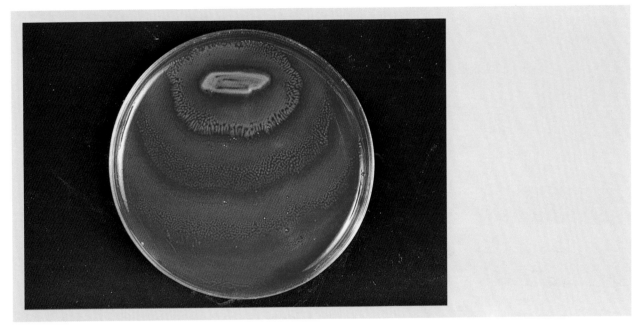

Figure 102 *Proteus mirabilis* swarming on blood agar. Pus from a polymicrobial pleural empyema may also contain facultative anaerobes (organisms which can grow both aerobically and anaerobically) such as staphylococci and enterobacteria. *Proteus*, *Escherichia coli* and *Klebsiella* are enterobacteria (coliforms) frequently cultured from pus, particularly in immunocompromised patients or those on intensive care units. Proteus swarms across blood agar, and this characteristic, together with its fishy odor, makes it easily recognizable in the clinical laboratory

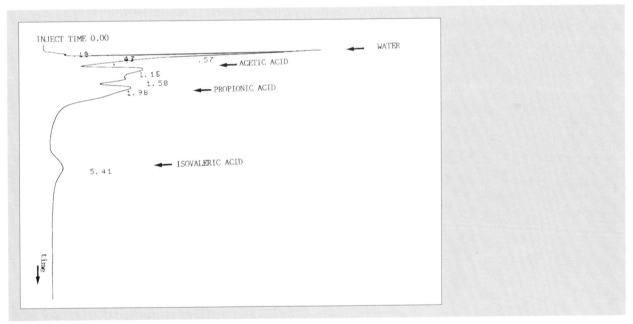

Figure 103 Gas–liquid chromatography chart demonstrating fatty acids produced by anaerobes in pus or broth culture. Anaerobes produce large numbers of fatty acids which account for the pungent odor of anaerobic pus. These can be detected in clinical specimens by gas–liquid chromatography (GLC), to provide a rapid diagnosis of anaerobic infection. Sometimes, the GLC tracing is characteristic of certain species. In this example, *Bacteroides fragilis* and *Peptostreptococcus* spp. are present

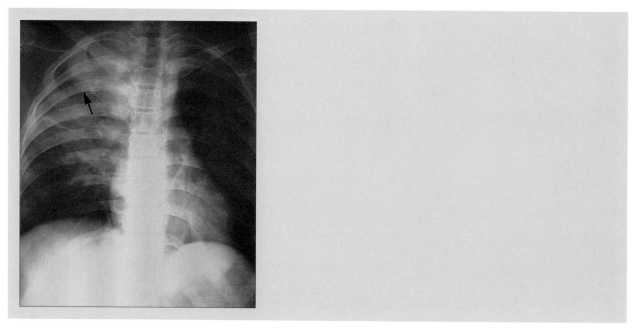

Figure 104 Actinomycosis. Chest radiograph shows consolidation of the right upper lobe and part of the lower lobe with an air bronchogram. Periosteal reaction is demonstrated along the lower border of the posterior ends of the right ribs (see arrow)

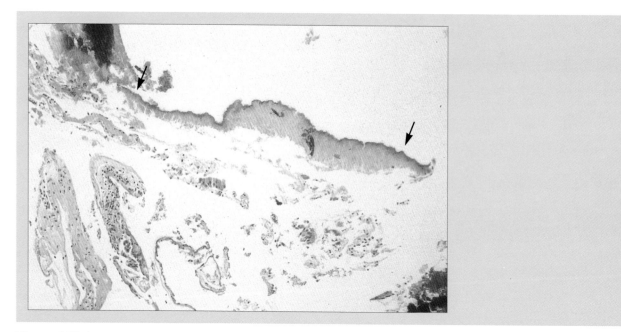

Figure 105 *Actinomyces israelii* in a section of lung. Hematoxylin & eosin × 800. A large plaque of organisms (arrows) has been biopsied. *Actinomyces* is a branching Gram-positive rod, closely related to *Nocardia*. It prefers anaerobic conditions for culture, although it is not a true anaerobe. It is slow growing in the laboratory and may need up to 2 weeks' incubation before colonies become visible. Specific culture methods are used and so the laboratory should be informed that actinomycosis is a possible diagnosis. *Actinomyces* spp. are found in the gingival crevice and in many cases pulmonary infection is thought to originate from dental sepsis. Pelvic actinomycotic infection associated with intrauterine contraceptive devices may also be a source of infection at other sites. Progressive destruction of soft tissue, cartilage and bone and sinus formation are classical features of untreated oral and pulmonary actinomycosis, but are rare

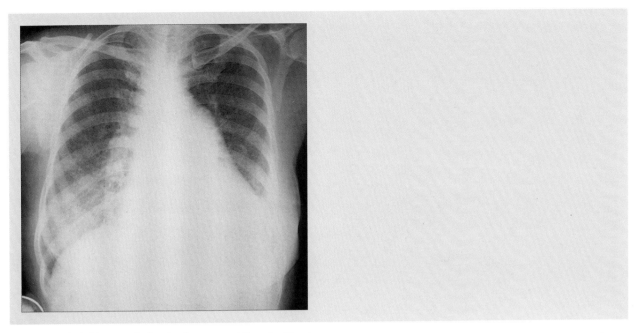

Figure 106 Schistosomiasis, also known as bilharzia. Chest radiograph confirms the diagnosis of pulmonary hypertension with prominent pulmonary vessels. Interstitial shadowing is visible throughout the lung fields

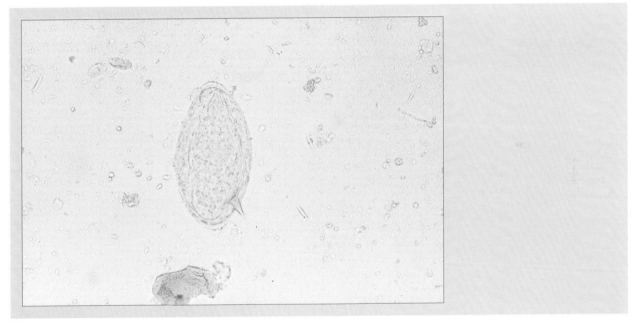

Figure 107 *Schistosoma mansoni* ovum. Wet mount preparation × 150. *Schistosoma* may cause chronic pulmonary symptoms from the embolization of ova released from the mature worm. Ova of schistosomes are normally detected in a centrifuged sample of terminal urine (*S. haematobium*, *S. japonicum*) or in a rectal biopsy (*S. mansoni*). The ova are identified by the position of the spine projecting from the ovum: *S. haematobium* (terminal); *S. japonicum* (rounded lateral); *S. mansoni* (pointed lateral). Schistosomiasis is acquired in fresh water in endemic areas when cercariae penetrate the skin of a new host. They migrate to the liver and lungs, develop into adult worms there and migrate a second time through the venous system to reach the bladder or portal venous plexi. The adult female, constantly fertilized by the male, releases ova that enter the urine or feces, depending on the species. These ova may also enter the systemic circulation. When in contact with fresh water, each ovum hatches a miracidium that penetrates a specific type of water snail and multiplies within it. After several weeks, cercariae are released which penetrate the skin of a new host

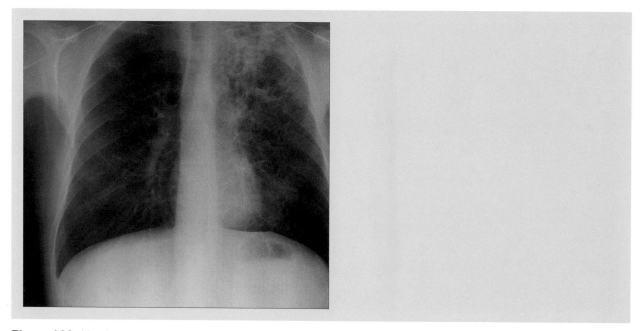

Figure 108 *Mycobacterium tuberculosis.* Chest radiograph shows bilateral upper lobe cavitation in post-primary infection

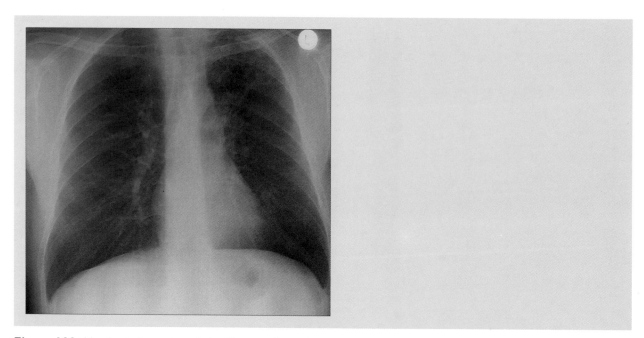

Figure 109 *Mycobacterium tuberculosis.* Chest radiograph of same patient as in Figure 108 shows residual fibrosis after 9 months of antituberculous treatment and corticosteroids for post-primary infection

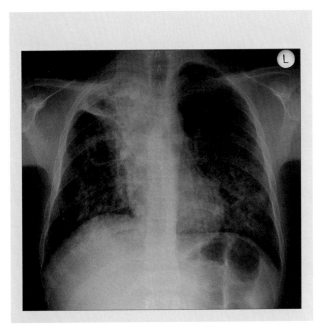

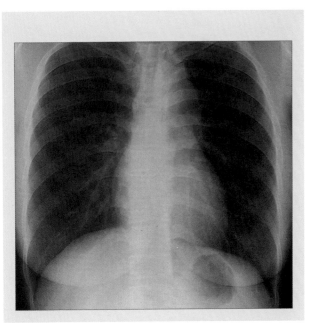

Figure 110 Diffuse pneumonia. Chest radiograph shows diffuse nodular shadowing throughout both lung fields with cavitation and collapse of the right upper lobe

Figure 111 Left hilar and paratracheal lymphadenopathy in a patient with tuberculosis infection. Chest radiograph

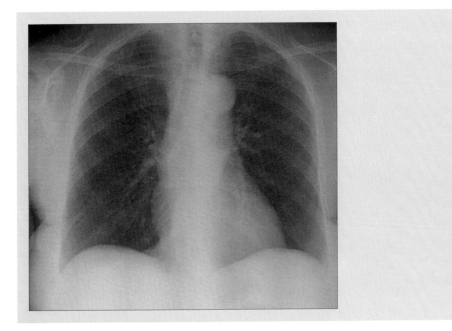

Figure 112 Miliary shadowing in a patient with tuberculosis. Chest radiograph shows 'millet seeds' of miliary shadowing

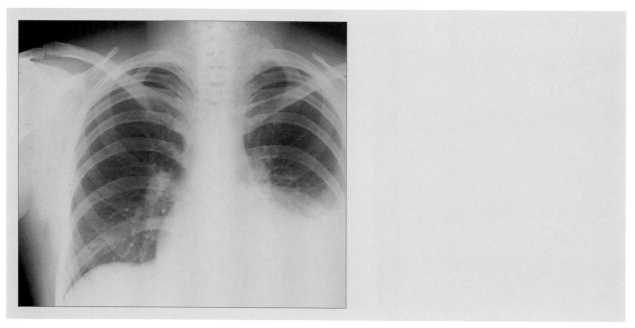

Figure 113 Tuberculous empyema. Chest radiograph shows left pleural effusion

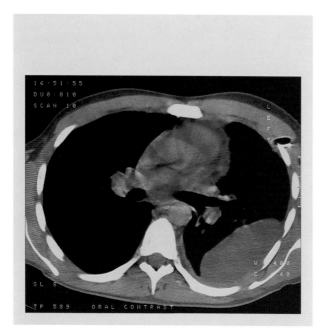

Figure 114 Tuberculous empyema. CT scan of thorax shows empyema with no pathology in the underlying lung

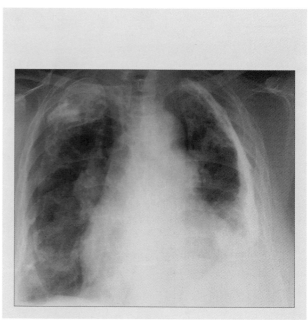

Figure 115 Old tuberculous empyema. Chest radiograph shows marked bilateral pleural calcification

Figure 116 Auramine stain. The auramine stain is a variation of the Ziehl–Neelsen stain and uses a fluorescent auramine dye instead of carbol fuschin. The slide is examined using an ultraviolet light microscope, and any acid-alcohol-fast bacilli will fluoresce. The advantage of this method lies in the greater prominence of the acid-alcohol-fast bacilli at lower microscopic power, and therefore larger fields of the slide smear can be examined

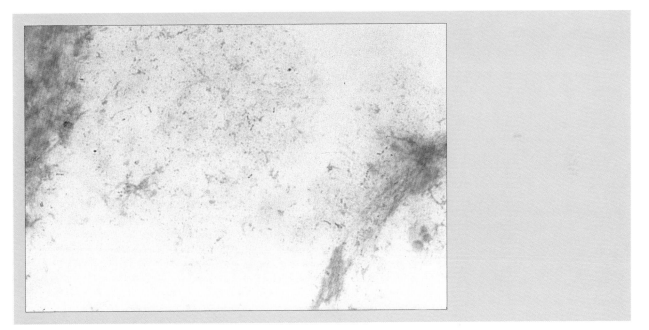

Figure 117 Ziehl–Neelsen stain of sputum showing acid-alcohol-fast bacilli × 800. In the Ziehl–Neelsen stain, a dried smear of a specimen or culture is treated with hot carbol fuschin (red), followed by hydrochloric acid with alcohol as the decolorization procedure, and then finally with a green/blue counterstain for a few seconds. Most bacteria are decolorized and appear blue (the color of the counterstain). *Mycobacterium* spp. is an acid-alcohol-fast bacillus, i.e. it retains the carbol fuschin stain and appears red. The Ziehl–Neelsen stain is of prime importance in the diagnosis of tuberculosis because acid-alcohol-fast bacilli seen in stained smears of sputum, bronchoalveolar lavage fluid, pus or other tissue are nearly always *Mycobacterium tuberculosis* or one of the other important mycobacteria. *M. tuberculosis* is long and thin, and, when present in large numbers, is arranged in bundles ('cords'). The *modified Ziehl–Neelsen stain* uses weaker acid for decolorization, and is used in the identification of organisms such as *Nocardia* and *Actinomyces*

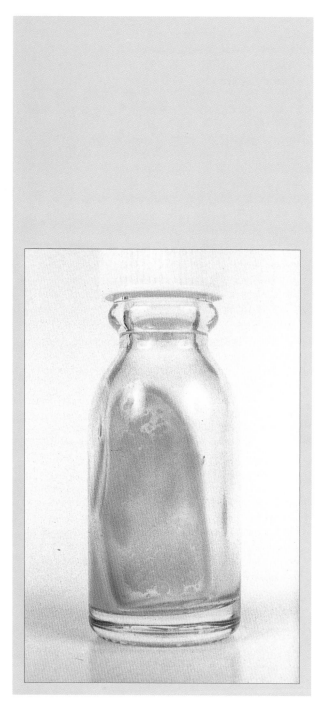

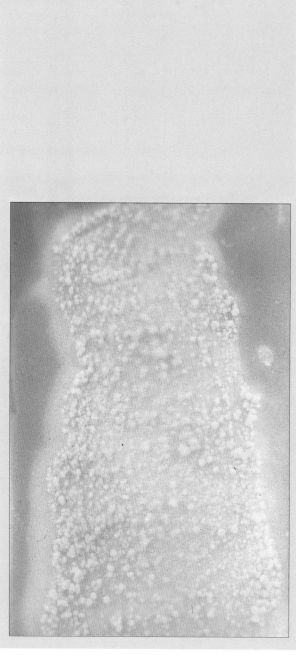

Figure 118 Lowenstein–Jensen slope growing *Mycobacterium tuberculosis*. Lowenstein–Jensen medium contains heated egg yolk, glycerol and malachite green; pyruvic acid can also be added to enhance growth of some species of mycobacteria. The medium is poured as a slope in a secure screw-capped bottle in order to prevent drying of the slope and to reduce the risk of laboratory-acquired infection from the culture. Many mycobacteria are very slow-growing; on a Lowenstein–Jensen slope, it can take 3–8 weeks for colonies to become visible. The colonies are typically described as 'rough (in appearance), tough (on manipulation with a wire loop) and buff (color)'

Figure 119 Lowenstein–Jensen slope (close view)

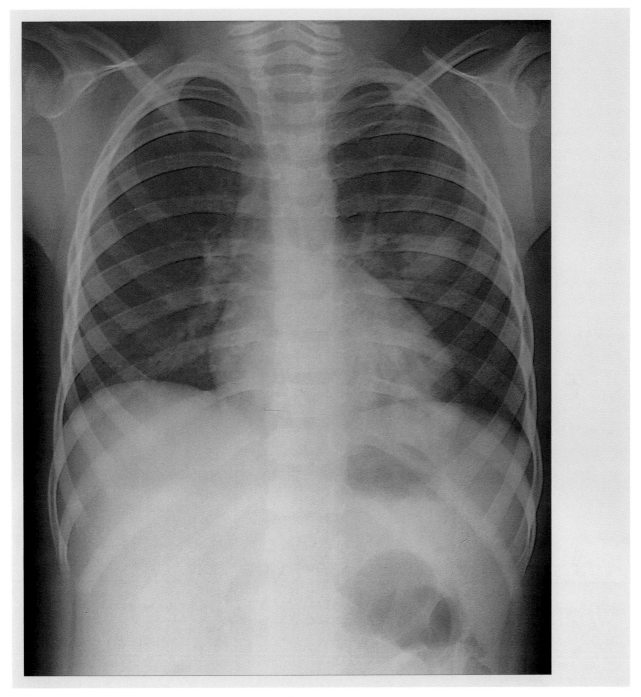

Figure 120 Pneumococcal infection in a child. Chest radiograph shows consolidation in the left mid-zone with right hilar lymphadenopathy

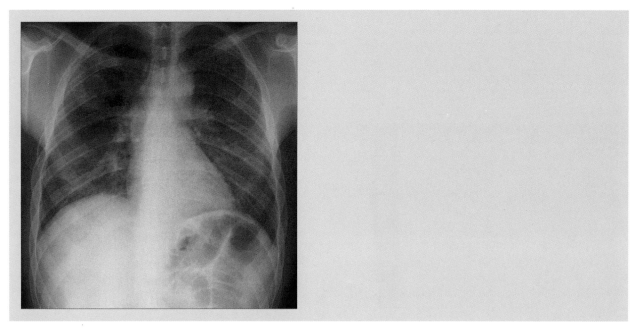

Figure 121 *Pneumocystis carinii* pneumonia. Chest radiograph

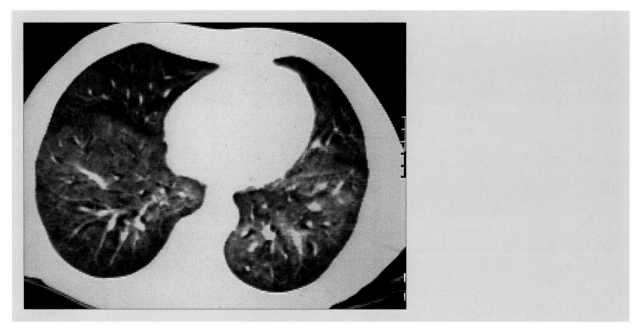

Figure 122 *Pneumocystis carinii* pneumonia. CT scan shows marked interstitial change within the lung parenchyma

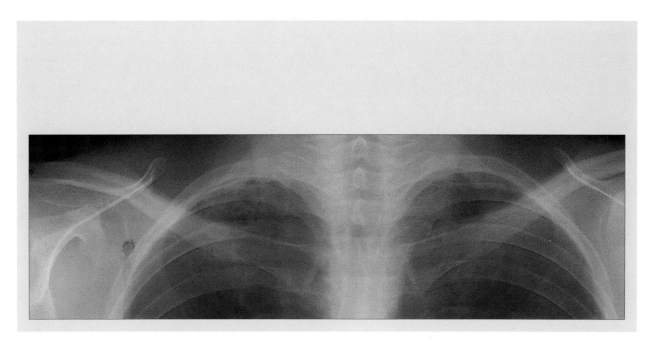

Figure 123 Atypical *Pneumocystis carinii* pneumonia. Chest radiograph shows bilateral apical cavitation in a patient with HIV infection

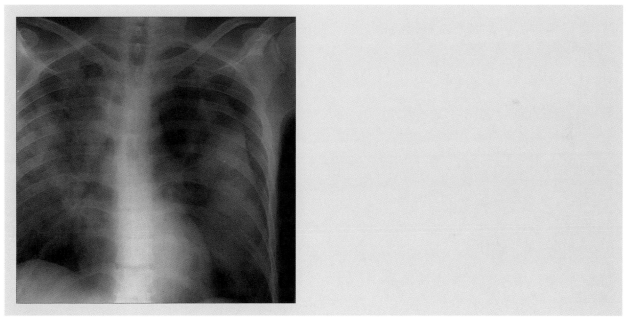

Figure 124 Chest radiograph of a patient with both *Pneumocystis carinii* and *Mycobacterium tuberculosis*. There is a left-sided pneumothorax

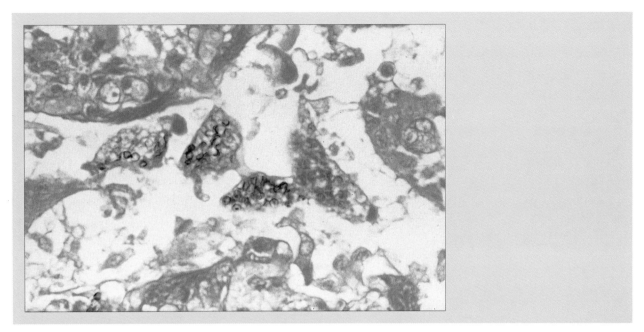

Figure 125 *Pneumocystis carinii:* Grocott silver stain of bronchoalveolar lavage fluid × 800. A silver stain or modified Giemsa stain will demonstrate *Pneumocystis carinii* in about 70–80% of patients with this infection. There is no *in vitro* culture method for *Pneumocystis*. Previously it was thought to be a protozoan but recently nucleic acid studies have shown it to be a fungus. A fluorescein-labelled monoclonal antibody is also available for staining the organism

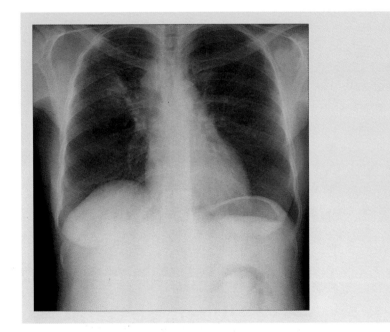

Figure 126 *Mycobacterium tuberculosis* pneumonia. Chest radiograph shows right upper zone consolidation with hilar lymphadenopathy typical of tuberculosis, with elevation of the right hemi-diaphragm indicative of underlying fibrosis

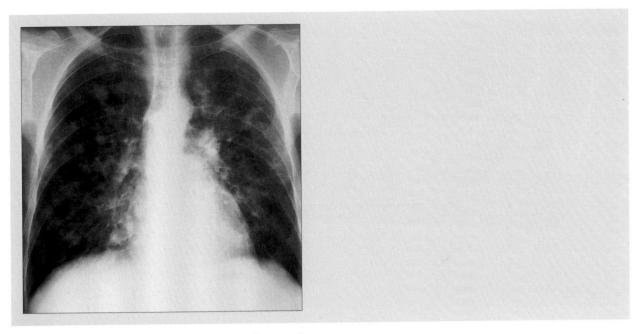

Figure 127 *Mycobacterium avium* complex. Chest radiograph

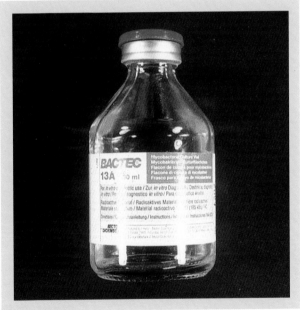

Figure 128 *Mycobacterium avium* complex: Ziehl–Neelsen stain of a culture × 800. The atypical bacteria such as *Mycobacterium avium* complex are often different in appearance from *M. tuberculosis*. *M. avium* complex is much shorter and fatter and cording (bundling of bacilli in groups) is not seen

Figure 129 Mycobacterial blood cultures. *Mycobacterium avium* complex may be cultured from the blood of AIDS patients using a mycobacterial blood culture system which detects production of CO_2 radiometrically (Bactec® Becton-Dickinson Ltd). The system can also be used as an enrichment medium to culture *M. tuberculosis* from clinical samples such as pleural fluid and other sites which are normally sterile

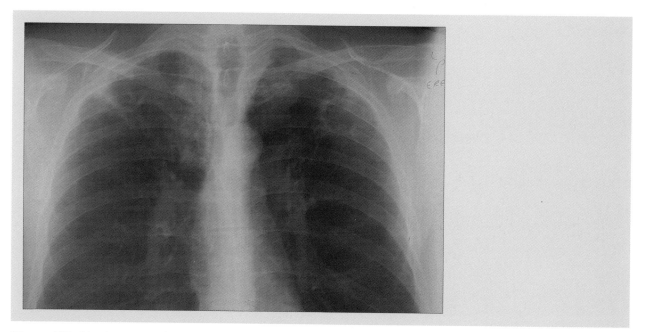

Figure 130 *Mycobacterium kansasii*. Chest radiograph shows bilateral cavitating apical shadowing

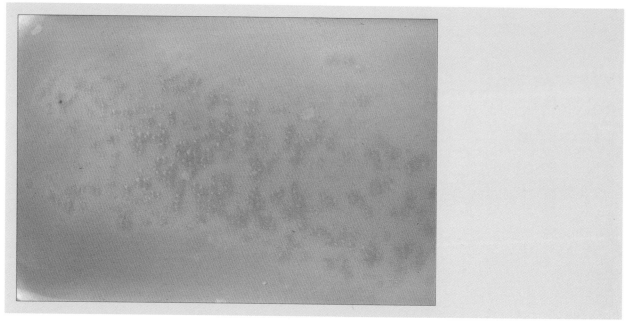

Figure 131 *Mycobacterium kansasii*: Lowenstein–Jensen slope. Cultures of certain species of 'atypical' mycobacteria produce pigment when exposed to light (photochro- mogens) or in the dark (scotochromogens). *Mycobacterium kansasii* is a photochromogen

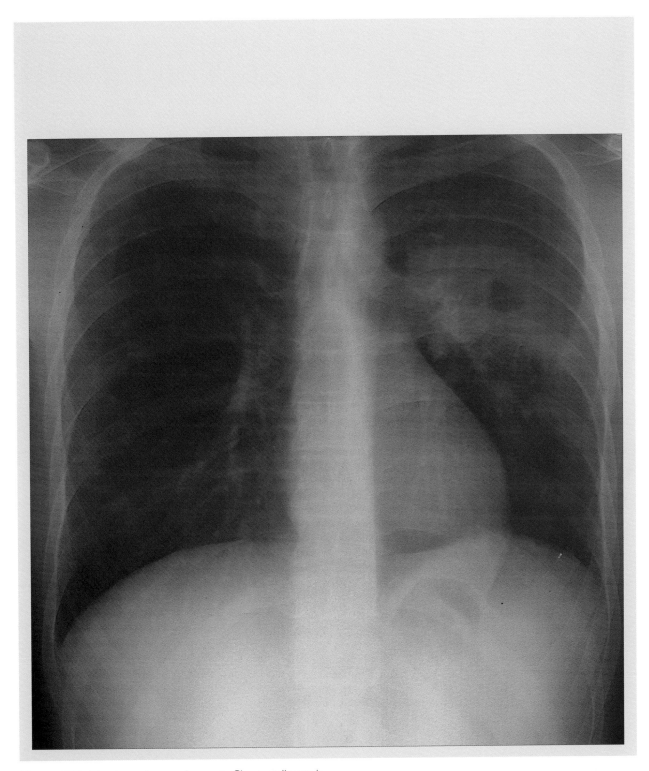

Figure 132 *Mycobacterium malmoensii.* Chest radiograph
shows cavitating mass in the left mid-zone with surrounding
parenchymal change but no node involvement

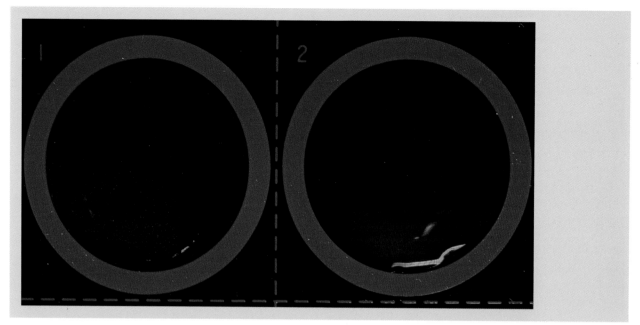

Figure 133 *Cryptococcus neoformans* antigen detection. *Cryptococcus* is a yeast surrounded by a large polysaccharide capsule. Cryptococcal capsular antigen can be detected in the blood of patients with lung or central nervous system infection. Latex particles coated with antibody to the capsular antigens are mixed with serum or cerebrospinal fluid. The left-hand sample (1) is positive for cryptococcal antigen. Cryptococcal antigen detection is sensitive and specific and provides a rapid result, and an antigen titer can be measured (the titer declines with successful therapy). Cryptococci can also be cultured in the laboratory on conventional media

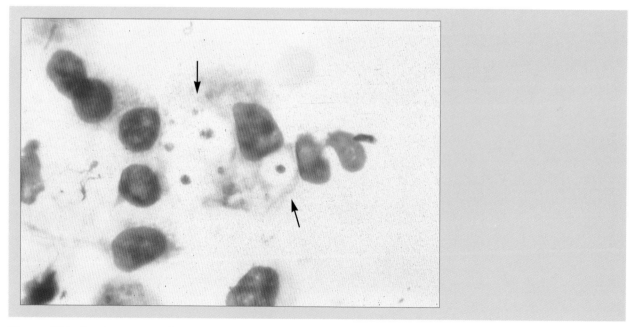

Figure 134 *Cryptococcus neoformans*: modified Giemsa stain × 1000. The yeasts (arrows), with their large capsules, can be seen within the macrophage. Photograph courtesy of Dr W. Keith Hadley, San Francisco General Hospital

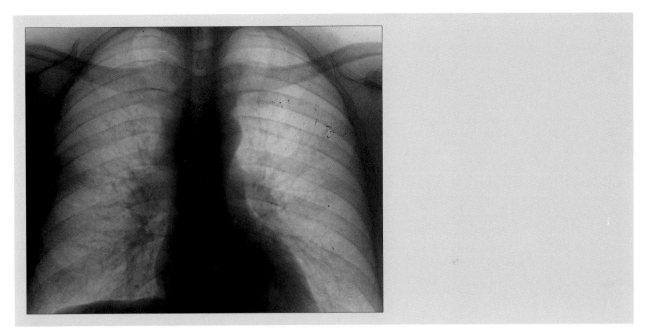

Figure 135 Disseminated coccidioidomycosis. Enlarged chest radiograph shows diffuse nodular infiltrates involving the entire lung field. Film courtesy of Dr Jeffery Klein, San Francisco General Hospital and Professor Phillip C. Hopewell, University of California, San Francisco

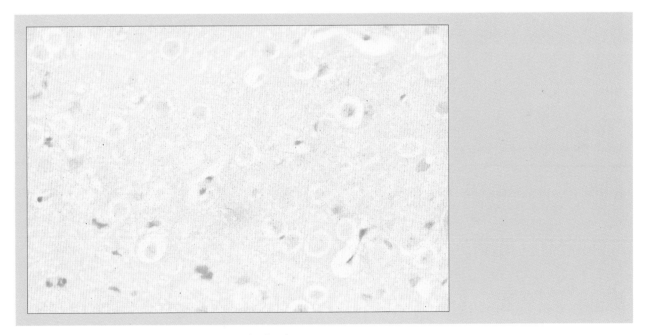

Figure 136 *Toxoplasma gondii* in mouse brain: hematoxyin & eosin × 500. Discrete toxoplasma cysts can be seen within the cortex. Pneumonitis may be a feature of disseminated toxoplasmosis, together with central nervous system infection, in either the immunocompromised host or infants with congenital toxoplasmosis

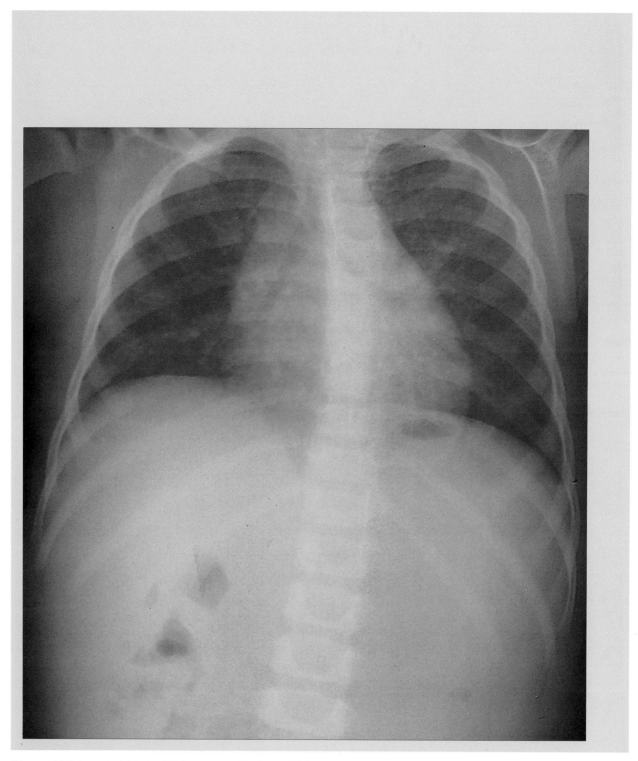

Figure 137 Lymphoid interstitial pneumonitis in a child. Chest radiograph shows bilateral interstitial disease and hilar lymphadenopathy

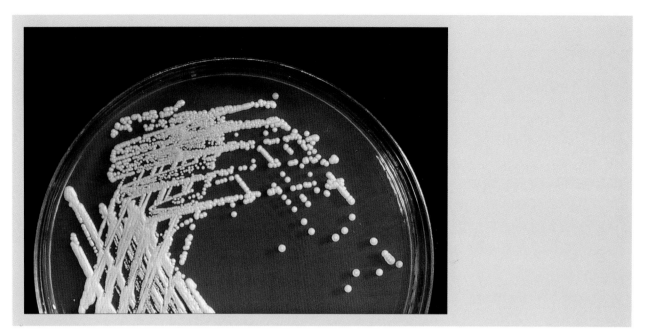

Figure 138 *Candida albicans* on Sabouraud's agar. *Candida* may be cultured from lower respiratory tract specimens but usually represents contamination from the oropharynx. Although candida pneumonia is relatively rare, concurrent isolation from bronchial lavage fluid and blood (or urine) would strongly suggest pulmonary infection. *Candida* is a yeast-like fungus which is readily grown on most types of agar. Sabouraud's agar is a selective medium for fungi. Detection of candida antigen in body fluids has been found to be a useful adjunct to the diagnosis of invasive candidiasis, in some centers

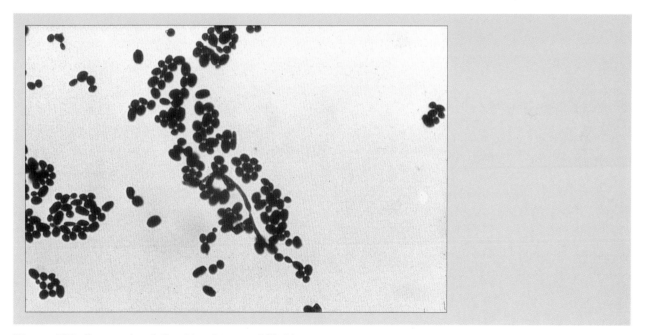

Figure 139 Gram stain of *Candida albicans* × 800. Yeast-like fungi such as *Candida* spp. can be seen on a Gram stain (although their cell wall is completely unlike that of Gram-positive bacteria). The yeasts replicate by budding and they form 'pseudohyphae' which are particularly prominent in specimens from clinical candida infections

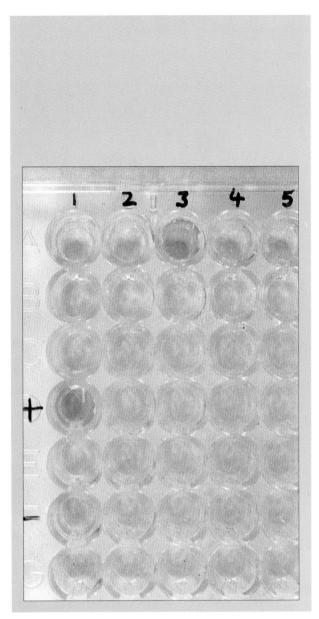

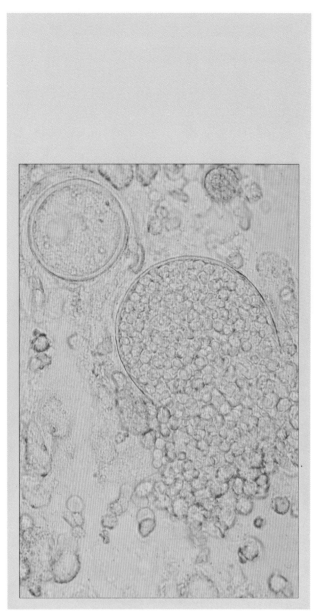

Figure 140 ELISA test for human immunodeficiency virus infection. Any patient with pneumonia likely to be caused by opportunist pathogens, and with known or suspected risk behavior for HIV infection, should be counselled about the need for an HIV antibody test. The enzyme-linked immunosorbent assay (ELISA) is the most common method of testing for antibodies to HIV types 1 and 2. HIV antigens bound to the microtiter plate are exposed to the patient's serum. After washing, an anti-human antibody labelled with enzyme is added to the well, and excess labelled antibody is washed off. A reagent which develops color (e.g. yellow or red) when exposed to the enzyme is then added. A positive antibody result (well 3) is indicated by the color change, which can be detected spectrophotometrically as well as visually. Positive and negative controls are included. A positive test is always confirmed by other methods, and tests for p24 antigen may also be performed

Figure 141 *Coccidioides immitis*: spherical disgorging endospores, in bronchoalveolar lavage fluid. Wet preparation × 1800. *Coccidioides immitis* is a dimorphic fungus found in soil in the south western United States, Central and South America. The diagnosis of coccidioidomycosis can be made by examining clinical specimens, mounted in potassium hydroxide solution. The organism can be cultured in the laboratory but extreme care must be taken as the cultures are highly infectious; sealed culture slopes and an exhaust protective cabinet must be used. Photograph courtesy of Dr W. Keith Hadley, San Francisco General Hospital

Section 3   Bibliography

Agostini, C., Zambello, R., Trentin, L., Poletti, V., Spiga, L., Gritti, F., Cipriani, A., Salmaso, L., Cadrobbi, P. and Semenzato, G. (1991). Prognostic significance of the evaluation of bronchoalveolar lavage cell populations in patients with HIV-1 infection and pulmonary involvement. *Chest*, **100**, 1601–6

Berman, L. A., (1991). Acute respiratory infections. *Infect. Dis. Clin. North Am.*, **5**, 319–36

Brewis, R. A. L., Gibson, G. J. and Geddes, D. M. (1990). *Respiratory Medicine*. (London: Balliere-Tindall)

Burman, L. A., Trollfors, B., Andersson, B., Henrichsen, J., Juto, P., Kallings, I., Lagergård, T., Möllby, R. and Norrby, R. (1991). Diagnosis of pneumonia by cultures, bacterial and viral antigen tests and serology with special reference to antibodies against pneumococcal antigens. *J. Infect. Dis.*, **163**, 1087–93

Campbell, H., Byass, P., Lamont, A. C., Forgie, I. M., O'Neill, K. P., Lloyd-Evans, N. and Greenwood, B. M. (1989). Assessment of clinical criteria for identification of severe acute lower respiratory tract infections in children. *Lancet*, **1**, 297–9

Cherian, T., John, T. J., Simoes, E., Steinhoff, M. C. and John, M. (1988). Evaluation of simple clinical signs for the diagnosis of acute lower respiratory tract infection. *Lancet*, **2**, 125–8

Derish, M. T., Kulhanjian, J. A., Frankel, L. R. and Smith, D. W. (1991). Value of bronchoalveolar lavage in diagnosing severe respiratory syncytial virus infections in infants. *J. Pediatr.*, **119**, 761–3

Donowitz, G. R. and Mandell, G. L. (1994). Acute pneumonia. In Mandell, G. L., Bennett, J. E. and Dolin, R. (eds.) *Principles and Practice in Infectious Diseases*. (New York: Churchill Livingstone)

Douglas, R. M. (1991). Acute respiratory infections in children in the developing world. *Semin. Respir. Infect.*, **6**, 217–24

Facklam, R. R. and Breiman, R. F. (1991). Current trends in bacterial respiratory pathogens. *Am. J. Med.*, **91**, 3–11S

Feuerstein, I. M., Archer, A., Pluda, J. M., Francis, P. S., Falloon, J., Masur, H., Pass, H. I. and Travis, W. D. (1990). Thin-walled cavities, cysts and pneumothorax in *Pneumocystis carinii* pneumonia: further observations with histopathologic correlations. *Radiology*, **174**, 697–702

Grainger, R. G. and Allison, D. J. (eds.) (1992). *Diagnostic Radiology*. (Edinburgh: Churchill Livingstone)

Heurlin, N., Elvin, K., Lidman, C., Lidman, K. and Lundbergh, P. (1990). Fiberoptic bronchoscopy and sputum examination for diagnosis of pulmonary disease in AIDS patients in Stockholm. *Scand. J. Infect. Dis.*, **22**, 659–64

Hietala, J., Uhari, M. and Tuokko, H. (1988). Antigen detection in the diagnosis of viral infections. *Scand. J. Infect. Dis.*, **20**, 595–9

Hoover, D. R., Graham, N. M., Bacellar, H., Schrager, L. K., Kaslow, R., Visscher, B., Murphy, R., Anderson, R. and Saah, A. (1991). Epidemiologic patterns of upper respiratory illness and *Pneumocystis carinii* pneumonia in homosexual men. *Am. Rev. Respir. Dis.*, **144**, 756–9

Kahn, F. W. and Jones, J. M. (1988). Analysis of bronchoalveolar lavage specimens from immunocompromised patients with a protocol applicable in the microbiology laboratory. *J. Clin. Microbiol.*, **26**, 1150–5

Marquette, C. H., Ramon, P., Courcol, R., Wallaert, B., Tonnel, A. B. and Voisin, C. (1988). Bronchoscopic protected catheter brush for the diagnosis of pulmonary infections. *Chest*, **93**, 746–50

Matthey, S., Nicholson, D., Ruhs, S., Alden, B., Knock, M., Schultz, K. and Schmuecker, A. (1992). Rapid detection of respiratory viruses by shell vial culture and direct staining by using pooled and individual monoclonal antibodies. *J. Clin. Microbiol.*, **30**, 540–4

Merrill, W., Marcy, T. A. and Reynolds, H. Y. (1988). Bronchoalveolar lavage: clinical role and quantitative assessment. *Respiration*, **54** (Suppl. 1), 3–8

Murphy, T. F. (1990). Molecular biology and respiratory disease. 6. Modern molecular biology and respiratory bacterial infections: a revolution on the horizon. *Thorax*, **45**, 552–9

Nohynek, H., Teppo, A. M., Laine, E., Leinonen, M. and Eskola, J. (1991). Serum tumor necrosis factor-alpha concentrations in children hospitalized for acute lower respiratory tract infection. *J. Infect. Dis.*, **163**, 1029–32

O'Doherty, M. J., Breen, D., Page, C., Barton, I. and Nunan, T. O. (1991). Lung 99mTc DTPA transfer in renal disease and pulmonary infection. *Nephrol. Dial. Transplant.*, **6**, 582–7

Pagliuca, A., Layton, D. M., Allen, S. and Mufti, G. J. (1988). Hyperinfection with strongyloides after treatment for adult T cell leukaemia-lymphoma in an African immigrant. *Br. Med. J.*, **297**, 1456

Pattyn, S. R., Provinciael, D., Lambrechts, R. and Ceuppens, P. (1991). Rapid diagnosis of viral respiratory infections. Comparison between immunofluorescence on clinical samples and immunofluorescence on centrifuged cell cultures. *Acta Clin. Belg.*, **46**, 7–12

Ramsey, B. W., Wentz, K. R., Smith, A. L., Richardson, M., Williams-Warren, J., Hedges, D. L., Gibson, R., Redding, G. J., Lent, K. and Harris, K. (1991). Predictive value of oropharyngeal cultures for identifying lower airway bacteria in cystic fibrosis patients. *Am. Rev. Respir. Dis.*, **144**, 331–7

Reuland, D. S., Steinhoff, M. C., Gilman, R. H., Bara, M., Olivares, E. G., Jabra, A. and Finkelstein, D. (1991). Prevalence and prediction of hypoxemia in children with respiratory infections in the Peruvian Andes. *J. Pediatr.*, **119**, 900–6

Salomon, H. E., Grandien, M., Avila, M. M., Pettersson, C. A. and Weissenbacher, M. C. (1989). Comparison of three techniques for detection of respiratory viruses in nasopharyngeal aspirates from children with lower acute respiratory infections. *J. Med. Virol.*, **28**, 159–62

Shure, D. (1989). Transbronchial biopsy and needle aspiration. *Chest*, **95**, 1130–8

Soderstrom, M., Hovelius, B., Prellner, K. and Schalen, C. (1990). Quantification of nasopharyngeal bacteria for diagnosis of respiratory tract infection in children. *Scand. J. Infect. Dis.*, **22**, 333–7

Stout, C., Murphy, M. D., Lawrence, S. and Julian, S. (1989). Evaluation of a monoclonal antibody pool for rapid diagnosis of respiratory viral infections. *J. Clin. Microbiol.*, **27**, 448–52

Strand, C. L. (1990). Role of the microbiology laboratory in the diagnosis of opportunistic infections in persons infected with human immunodeficiency virus. *Arch. Pathol. Lab. Med.*, **114**, 277–83

Takimoto, S., Grandien, M., Ishida, M. A., Pereira, M. S., Paiva, T. M., Ishimaru, T., Makita, E. M. and Martinez, C. H. (1991). Comparison of enzyme-linked immunosorbent assay, indirect immunofluorescence assay, and virus isolation for detection of respiratory viruses in nasopharyngeal secretions . *J. Clin. Microbiol.*, **29**, 470–4

Terpstra, W. J., Groeneveld, K., Eijk, P. P., Geelen, L. J., Schoone, G. J., ter-Schegget, J., van-Nierop, J. C., Griffioen, R. W. and van Alphen, L. (1988). Comparison of two nonculture techniques for detection of *Haemophilus influenzae* in sputum. *In situ* hybridization and immunoperoxidase staining with monoclonal antibodies. *Chest*, **94** (Suppl. 2), 126–9S

Weldon-Linne, C. M., Rhone, D. P. and Bourassa, R. (1990). Bronchoscopy specimens in adults with AIDS. Comparative yields of cytology, histology and culture for diagnosis of infectious agents. *Chest*, **98**, 24–8

Wood, B. P. (1989). Pediatric lung disease. *Curr. Opin. Radiol.*, **1**, 557–62

Index